Jesus came so that we might enjoy an abundant life. Through the vibrant palette of His creation, God has provided a wide spectrum of natural resources that promote health and healing in our bodies, and my friend Teri Secrest has found a well of insight into one of these pathways to well-being: essential oils. In her book, Teri unpacks the biblical backdrop for many of these oils as she shares remarkable stories of God's goodness being displayed through the use of essential oils. *Essential Oils: God's Extravagant Provision for Your Health* will take you on an eye-opening journey and help you to explore more of God's heart for His children.

—*Dr. Ché Ahn*
President, Harvest International Ministry
Founding and Senior Pastor, HROCK Church, Pasadena, CA
International Chancellor, Wagner University

Essential Oils: God's Extravagant Provision for Your Health strategically combines knowledge and experience from one of the top women entrepreneurs in the world. It is biblical. It is solid. Yet, it is also holistic and integrated. It is my delight to endorse this groundbreaking book by a disciple of the Lord Jesus Christ and a personal dear friend. Don't just read this book—apply the truths!

—*Dr. James W. Goll*
Founder, God Encounters Ministries
Author, Speaker, Communications Trainer, and Recording Artist

I have known Teri Secrest for many years, and I have watched how her loving and caring personality warms the hearts of those around her. I have really enjoyed her thoughtful insight into life and the things that matter.

Although my husband, D. Gary Young, discovered that essential oils offered wonderful physical benefits to both man and animals, he also believed that the healing of emotional and spiritual problems of God's children was the foundation for physical healin~~~~~~~~~~~~~~~~~~~~~convinced that essential oils could uplift and elevate consciou~~~~~~~~~~~~~~~~~~~~~~~oser to achieving their highest potential.

D1505166

Teri connected immediately to Gary's teachings and wanted to know more. She has done her own research and made her own discoveries that have made her path very certain. She has a strong knowing of who she is, which comes from her connection to God and the spiritual things of this world, which is a passionate force in her life.

Many people wonder about their purpose and the path they should follow. When we are physically and emotionally healthy, our minds become unclouded and we can more easily determine our path.

Teri's desire is to help people come to an understanding that living in a clean environment and eating wholesome food is part of God's direction to his children. It is fascinating to read in the Scriptures how essential oils were used anciently and to realize that God's instruction then is just as powerful for us today. The pure essence of Mother Nature, the essential oils enhance our awareness and give us strength and motivation to follow our dreams.

Teri has written about so many facets of life in a loving and understandable way, which gives that little push to help people move in the right direction. It is interesting how she brings all the parts together to create a whole way of living for a productive, healthy, and abundant life.

—*Mary Young*
CEO, Young Living Essential Oils

Essential Oils: God's Extravagant Provision for Your Health by Teri Secrest combines insight into many health-related issues and knowledge of precious oils with a kind and joyous nature to provide you with a warm introduction to the power of essential oils. She also shares many of her own healing experiences with essential oils to illustrate their power and usefulness. I know you will enjoy her book and greatly benefit from reading it.

—*Joan Hunter*
Author/Healing Evangelist
TV Host, *Miracles Happen!*

There is an anointing of joy that accompanies this book as it becomes apparent that *Essential Oils* is a display of the goodness and kindness of God to his people. Teri shines light on a very important subject that only receives a brief glimpse as we read the Scriptures.

You will realize why the wise men from the East include frankincense and myrrh as a gift to honor the Christ child. You will begin to appreciate the healing power of these oils, both physically and emotionally. You will go on a personal journey with Teri as she discovered this unique gift from God.

Thank you, Teri, for writing this beautiful book. I am challenged, not only to continue using these precious oils, but to look again into the Scriptures to understand a deeper expression of God's love and favor towards us.

Essential Oils is easy to read and understand, delightful, and written from the heart.

—*Dr. Royree Jensen*
Harvest International Ministry, Women on the Frontlines
Pastor, River of Life Church, Brisbane, Australia

This is a must read for anyone who wants to burn brightly without burning out. This book is a gift to all of us from Teri Secrest, a veteran leader who will coach you to a life of God-intended purpose and destiny.

—*Leif Hetland*
President, Global Mission Awareness
Author, *Called to Reign*

Teri Secrest's book, *Essential Oils: God's Extravagant Provision for Your Health*, brings the romance and intrigue of essential oils and blends it with everyday uses. This is not a technical book; it is a beautiful history wrapped in the elegance essential oils deserve, built upon a foundation of rock-solid research. Every essential oil user should own this book.

—*Beverly Banks*
Writer/Producer, *Ancient Secrets of Essential Oils*

Teri Secrest is a champion in bringing out hidden truths of how God has provided yet another way for us to walk in health. We know God wants us healthy. Teri expounds on 3 John 1:2: *"Beloved, I pray that in all respects you may prosper and be in good health, just as your soul prospers"* (NASB). God wants and has provided us avenues to become healthy in all aspects of our lives.

For some of us, essential oils are a new or a relatively new concept. Reading the insights Teri has gleaned from the Bible of oil's role in securing our physical, emotional, and spiritual wellbeing is mesmerizing! There are so many biblical examples and references that many of us have just skipped over, but they are there and there for a reason! God wants to show us how to live in health. And then there are the practical benefits provided by Teri's relentless study on the subject. Proverbs 25:2 says, *"It is the glory of God to conceal a matter, but the glory of kings is to search out a matter"* (NASB). That is exactly what Teri has done for us. She has searched it out.

Teri is living out and experiencing firsthand the results of what she shares in this book. We recommend it to you. You will experience an additional way that God has provided for us to live life in health!

—*Alan and Carol Koch*
Founding Pastors, Christ Triumphant Church, Koch Ministries

Riveting, inspiring, and beautifully written, this book is a must read! Teri provides a powerful, inspiring message of how essential oils can revitalize and strengthen your body, mind, and spirit. She has a way of bringing her life experiences into her teachings of the practical benefits of essential oils and helping you understand they are truly gifts from God. As Teri guides you through this book, filled with the tools needed to live a significant life, she provides an education with clever humor throughout.

—*Lata L. Lovell*
CEO, Landmarks of Eureka Springs, LLC
Queen Anne Estate, Eureka Springs, AR

If you have ever desired to prosper in body, soul, and health just like 3 John 1:2 tells us, then this book is for you. Teri's new book, *Essential Oils: God's*

Extravagant Provision for Your Health, grabs you in the introduction with a question that hits the heart like a one-two power punch: If I keep doing what I'm doing today, how healthy will I be five years from now?

If answering this question brings more fear and frustration than hope and excitement, this book is for you. Teri shows us an easy path to health by using essential oils. I have used essential oils for years and I did not know the deep truths revealed in this book. And the most amazing part is it's easy to follow and easy to do. I would go so far as to say if you desire to live a healthy, active life today as well as the decades ahead, then you simply must take the time to read this book and do what it says to do. Before your very eyes, you will see your body, soul, and health begin to prosper.

—Julie Meyer
Into the River Ministries
Author, *Singing the Scriptures*
On Staff, Healing Rooms Apostolic Center, Santa Maria, CA

Teri Secrest is a voice you will be blessed to hear and her book, *Essential Oils: God's Extravagant Provision for Your Health*, contains words you will be advantaged to read. This is an influence you will be touched by and changed for the better.

—Dr. Jack Taylor
President, Dimensions Ministries, Melbourne, FL

I am forever indebted to Teri for the wisdom and encouraging strength she has imparted to me to learn of God's garden of oils.

—Janet McBride
Author, *Scriptural Essence*

Teri Secrest radiates with integrity, courage, humility, and confidence. I'm excited about this intriguing new book and I look forward to opening my heart and testing the applications.

—Pastor Michael Sullivant
CEO, Life Model Works

The ever-increasing amount of industrialized and commercialized foods being promulgated across this country have had increasing negative impacts on our health. Kingdom health is extremely important to Teri and as a wellness coach, her passion has emerged from teacher to writer. Her latest book, *Essential Oils: God's Extravagant Provision for Your Health*, will help you create a pathway to perfect health and will enable you to influence others.

—*Joshua Mills*
Author, *Moving in Glory Realms and Seeing Angels*

ESSENTIAL
Oils

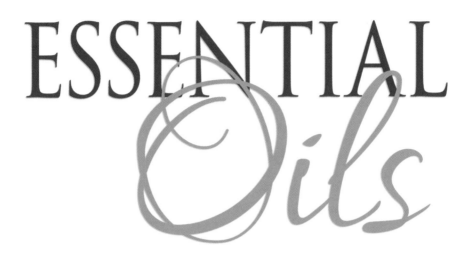

God's Extravagant Provision
for Your Health

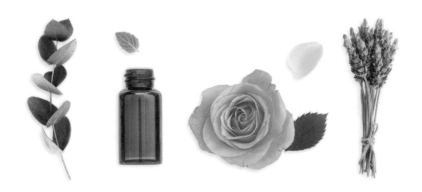

TERI SECREST

WHITAKER
HOUSE

This book is not intended to provide medical advice or to take the place of medical advice and treatment from your personal physician. Readers are advised to consult their own doctors or other qualified health professionals regarding the treatment of their medical problems. Neither the publisher nor the author takes any responsibility for any possible consequences from any treatment, action, or application of medicine, supplement, herb, or preparation to any person reading or following the information in this book. If readers are taking prescription medications, they should consult with their physicians and not take themselves off medicines to start supplementation without the proper supervision of a physician.

ESSENTIAL OILS
God's Extravagant Provision for Your Health

Teri Secrest
www.TeriSecrest.com

ISBN: 978-1-64123-329-3 • eBook ISBN: 978-1-64123-330-9
Printed in the United States of America
© 2019 by Teri Secrest

Whitaker House
1030 Hunt Valley Circle
New Kensington, PA 15068
www.whitakerhouse.com

Library of Congress Cataloging-in-Publication Data
Names: Secrest, Teri, 1953- author.
Title: Essential oils : God's extravagant provision for your health / Teri
   Secrest.
Description: New Kensington, PA : Whitaker House, [2019] | Includes
   bibliographical references and index. | Summary: "Provides information
   on the use of essential oils for health issues, romance, pets,
   fragrance, and cooking, as well as biblical accounts and the author's
   personal experiences and recipes"— Provided by publisher.
Identifiers: LCCN 2019024352 (print) | LCCN 2019024353 (ebook) | ISBN
   9781641233293 (hardcover) | ISBN 9781641233309 (ebook)
Subjects: LCSH: Essences and essential oils—Therapeutic use. | Essences
   and essential oils—Physiological effect. | Aromatherapy.
Classification: LCC RM666.A68 S387 2019 (print) | LCC RM666.A68 (ebook) |
   DDC 615.3/219—dc23
LC record available at https://lccn.loc.gov/2019024352
LC ebook record available at https://lccn.loc.gov/2019024353

1 2 3 4 5 6 7 8 9 10 11 **WH** 26 25 24 23 22 21 20 19

DEDICATION

This book is dedicated to the late D. Gary Young; his wife, Mary; and sons, Jacob and Josef.

As the father of modern-day essential oils distillation, D. Gary Young invested his mind, his heart, and all of his resources into the lifelong study and research on the value of essential oils for optimal health. As he discovered new plants and the value of their oil in the far corners of the earth, D. Gary Young lived in tireless dedication to teach others what he learned.

Mary Young stood by Gary's side through every joy and trial. Some might say she is the reason he often had super-human endurance! The love between this couple has inspired thousands.

Jacob and Josef, though still in their teens, already begin to carry the torch of hope that their father lit twenty-five years ago.

Although I have studied with others around the world, D. Gary Young was my greatest mentor, sometimes a father figure, and always a loyal friend. Because of what I have learned from his teachings, our family lives a healthy, strong, vibrant, and joyful life. With gratitude and love, I now share this knowledge with you. May this book fully honor the life and legacy of D. Gary Young by showing how you, too, can live a strong, healthy, and vibrant life!

—Teri Secrest

Diffuser Recipes

CONTENTS

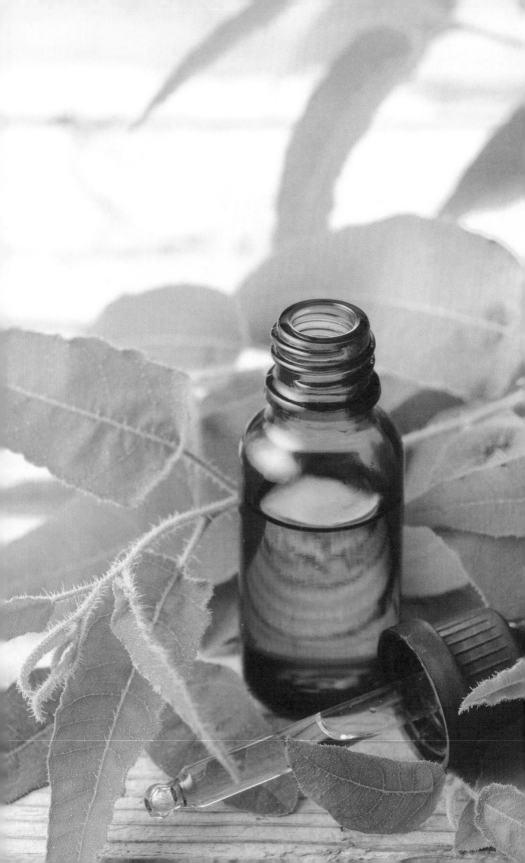

FOREWORD

I want to introduce you to the author of this book: my friend Teri Secrest. I have known Teri for a number of years and have enjoyed both her passion for the Lord and her heart to serve people. She has empowered many to enjoy optimum health over the years through her role as a health and wellness coach. Teri is an extremely generous woman and she would never want the knowledge and understanding that she obtained through her years of research and experience to remain solely with her. For as long as I have known her, she has been deeply passionate to see all people enjoy a life filled with vibrant health and happiness. As a result, she has committed her life to this cause.

Through her seminars, books, resources, personal coaching and essential oil products, she has given valuable, life-transforming insight to many. I personally did not know anything about essential oils until Teri came into my life. I knew that the Bible spoke a lot about oils, but had not considered the specific use of them in my life to enhance health and healing until Teri explained the benefit of them to me.

At the time I was initially introduced to the use of essential oils, I was fighting a cold and sore throat. Some specific oils were recommended that I breathe in and ingest. Within hours, the symptoms lifted. I also discovered that a little peppermint oil helped to awaken me during the day if I felt a little "brain fog" and that oil of lavender helped me relax at night. I loved that the oils were natural and promoted health in an easy and practical way.

Teri is one of the most genuine people you will meet. As a successful businesswoman, I have seen her equally value, help, and support both pauper and prince. She has stayed in my home, travelled with me, and labored with me in seminars and conferences, but she is always, consistently, loving well—what you see is what you get!

In this book, Teri shares some of her research discoveries, personal experiences, and testimonies of others. She offers the reader some valuable insights and practical tips for living a healthy life. Teri's positive outlook, her optimistic approach to challenges, and her joy-filled personality and child-like faith are refreshing.

I believe you will enjoy this book.

—*Patricia King*
Founder, Patricia King Ministries

PREFACE:
A LIFELONG MYSTERY SOLVED

It's Christmas Eve and billowing drifts of snow are racing across the frozen waters of Clear Lake. My brother, three sisters, and I are scrambling to get our best clothes on, just in time to pile into our slightly worn station wagon and head to midnight Mass.

As the youngest of five children, it was hard to pay attention through the entire Mass. But during the Christmas season, the one thing I never missed was when the priest read the story of the wise men giving gold, frankincense, and myrrh to the Christ child! That mesmerized me as somehow, I knew they must have been great treasures.

Have you ever wondered why the wise men brought frankincense and myrrh for the baby Jesus? As a curious and highly enthusiastic child, I asked everyone. But no one could answer my question. So I grew up thinking it was just some nice fairytale...but I never stopped wondering.

Fast forward to thirty years later; I was a health and wellness coach giving a lecture on the benefits of walking and healthy eating at the Salt Palace in Salt Lake City, Utah. Afterward, the late D. Gary Young walked up to me, introduced himself, and told me he really enjoyed my lecture. After talking with him about health for a few minutes, he said, "Teri, would you like to come to my lecture?" I replied, "Sure. What are you speaking on today, sir?"

Imagine my shock when he said he was giving a talk on frankincense and myrrh and his conviction that they are the missing link to natural health today. With a pounding heart, I replied, "Yes, sir, I would love to come to your lecture." *Finally*, I thought, *I am going to solve the mystery that has been in my heart for all these years!*

As Young started his talk, he pulled out his Bible and began to read verse after verse, from Genesis to Revelation, that referenced specific plant oils, now known as essential oils. He spoke about the third day of creation and how all of the trees, shrubs, plants, and flowers are God's provision for our physical and emotional health. As I listened, the answer to my life-long mystery unfolded before my eyes: this "liquid gold," these tiny drops of oil, were part of God's great plan from the foundation of the world to keep His children healthy in body, soul, and spirit.

I had such a powerful reaction to this new knowledge that I was literally hanging on to my chair. Thankfully, no one was watching me. I thought, *Teri, get a hold of yourself.*

Afterward, as I thanked Young for his astounding teaching, he placed something in my hand. "Here," he said, "you may need this one day." I

Lavende

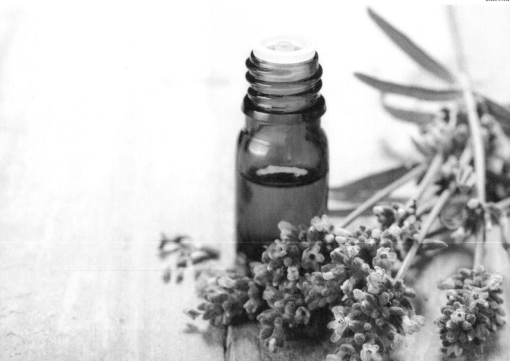

thanked him profusely and made my departure, as he had many other people waiting to talk with him. When I opened my hand, there was a bottle of lavender essential oil.

The only thing I knew about lavender oil was that several perfumes I had seen in Europe included it as an ingredient. (I had been blessed to live in Paris for two years.) So I thought Young had given it to me as a perfume. Being a very busy mother of two children with our third child on the way, I took my bottle of lavender oil and lovingly placed it in the front row of my pantry shelf, thinking I would learn more about it as soon as I had some free time.

On my very next trip to the bookstore, I went to the help desk and asked where I could find books on essential oils. The lady smiled kind of funny and said she had no idea what I was talking about, but she didn't think they had any books in the store like that. From the look on her face, I think she was expecting me to pull out a crystal ball at any minute. I soon discovered that virtually no information was available on essential oils, nor was there any information about essential oils in biblical history.

I pondered what I had learned for months. While the mystery about frankincense and myrrh was finally solved for me, it was months before I discovered why I had been given the bottle of lavender oil that day.

This sparked my twenty-three-year quest to learn about essential oils, a quest that has taken me to the far corners of the world—to Oman, Croatia, France, the Philippines, Israel, and other countries.

My purpose in writing this book is to inspire you with the mystery, the romance, and the ageless intrigue of essential oils. My hope is that you experience the Father's love as He continually lavishes His children with these exquisite essential oils and that this rich biblical history comes alive in your spirit. I also hope you will see how miraculous your body is and how it's designed to heal itself when given proper nourishment and support.

As you gain this understanding, I believe you will change the next generation, as you will know the hidden secrets of these biblical plants and how to incorporate them into your everyday life.

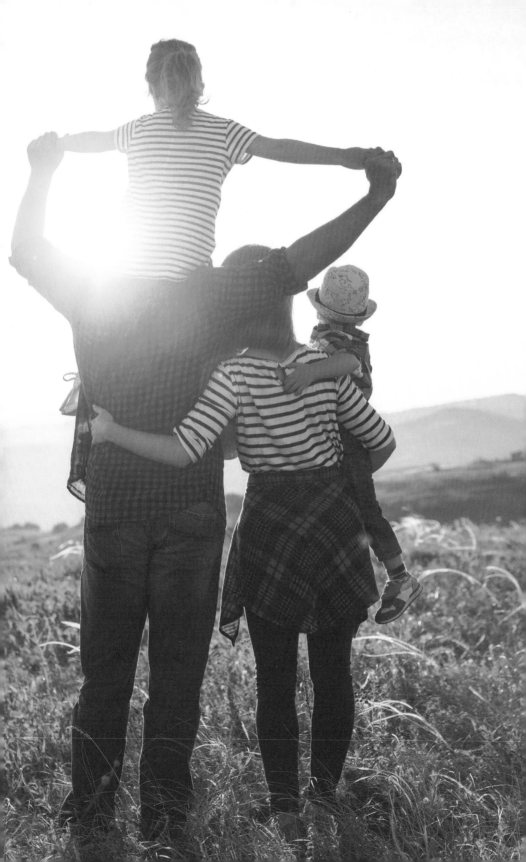

INTRODUCTION:
THE STATE OF HEALTH
IN AMERICA

A sk yourself these questions:

If I keep doing what I'm doing today, how healthy will I be five years from now?

When was the last time I felt absolutely fantastic, excited about life, full of energy, and jumped out of bed in the morning?

As a wellness coach, I ask my new clients questions like these. Some tell me they haven't felt fantastic for ten years—even twenty. Friend, that's not living. The good news is you live in a body that is designed to heal. Think about that for a minute: when you provide your body with the right food, water, movement, and sunshine it needs, it will perform miracles of healing every day. If you don't wake up feeling great, it's time to make some simple, easy changes so your body can begin operating at optimal levels and serve you as it is intended to do.

The following statistics opened my eyes to the seriousness of our national health and why it's vital that we make changes now.

Statistics Are Staggering

+ Approximately one in five cancer deaths, or 18 percent, are attributable to the combined effects of excess weight, alcohol consumption, poor nutrition, and a sedentary lifestyle.[1]

+ Seven of the top ten leading causes of death in the United States are due to chronic diseases such as type 2 diabetes, heart disease, and obesity. Treating people with these diseases accounts for 86 percent of the health care costs in the U.S.[2]

+ In 2015, an estimated 27 to 29 million Americans had type 2 diabetes.[3] Yet the Centers for Disease Control and Prevention estimates that *one-fourth* of all Americans with diabetes don't even know they have it.

+ More than one-third of American children eat fast food on any given day.[4] Studies directly link fast-food consumption to increased calorie intake, weight gain, and elevated risk for diabetes.[5]

+ Four out of five Americans are more than thirty pounds overweight, according to the National Center for Health Statistics. The rate of childhood obesity has *tripled* since 1980.[6]

+ According to the World Health Organization, approximately 300 million people are living with depression, up 18 percent since 2005.[7]

+ During years 2011 through 2014, about one in eight Americans ages twelve and older reported taking antidepressants in the previous month.[8] Antidepressant use increased nearly 65 percent between 1999 and 2014.

Friend, these facts are riveting! This is not what God desires for you.

God Wants Us to Enjoy Good Health

We live in a society where an ever-increasing amount of industrialized foods are being sold and eaten, which has greatly affected our health. The consequences of poor eating, obesity, and inactivity are epidemic levels of

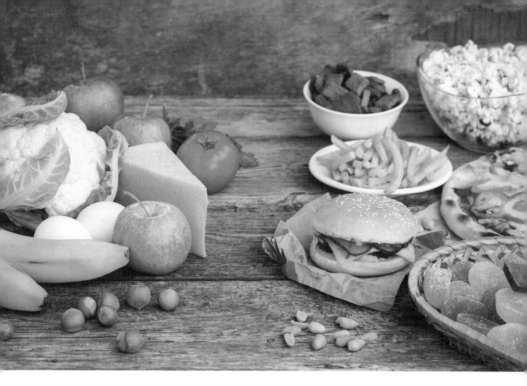

chronic disease. The tragedy is that most of these diseases are preventable or curable with better nutrition and more activity.

This is your opportunity to learn what's at stake and take a leadership role in your family's health.

With the average American family now consisting of two working parents, the notion of having three home-cooked meals a day, even on weekends, is a foreign concept. My heart really goes out to families who are trying to juggle the demands of real life in the twenty-first century. But fast food and prepacked food often causes our children to suffer from imbalances in their bodies that were once rare.

No loving parent would ever intentionally poison or neglect their child. Yet many doctors believe that type 2 diabetes and obesity are directly related to eating at fast-food restaurants day after day and purchasing low-quality foods laden with chemicals and additives.

This is God's plan for you:

Beloved, I pray that in all respects you may prosper and be in good health, just as your soul prospers.   (3 John 1:2 NASB)

Imagine standing before heaven's gatekeeper and being told, "You know, you were not due here for another twenty years. Your mansion may not be ready yet. Just a minute, I'd better go check." Wow. Wouldn't that be a terrible state of affairs?

God has great plans for you, something spectacular you came here to do, so I will do my part to make sure you stay here and fulfill your destiny.

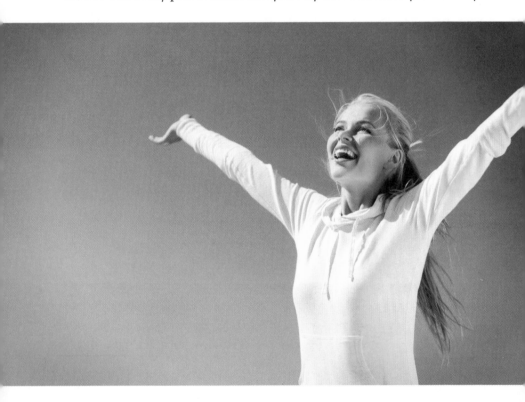

Making positive life changes takes a willing heart and a teachable spirit. Are you teachable? If you are feeling stubborn about changing some of your habits, consider this: if we could eat anything we wanted at any time, we would not be in the national health situation we are in. We are meant to experience joy in this life and we need to feel good to do that.

We know that our mind, our will, and our emotions reside in the soul. The Bible promises we will *"be in good health, just as [our] soul prospers."* The depression epidemic resides in the wounding of our souls. We must heal our souls to be totally well. In this book, you will learn the power of breathing God's plant oils for the healing of your mind, your will, and your emotions, so your soul may be free to soar again.

The enemy of your soul has other plans for you.

> *The thief comes only to steal and kill and destroy; I came that they may have life, and have it abundantly.*   (John 10:10 NASB)

Jesus came so that you might have life and have it more abundantly. It's time to think higher. You've got to tell the enemy where to go and believe in the goodness of God and His love for you. His great plans for you include hope and a future.

> *"For I know the plans I have for you," declares the LORD, "plans to prosper you and not to harm you, plans to give you hope and a future."*   (Jeremiah 29:11 NIV)

My goal in writing this book is to show you God's extravagant and lavish provision for your health, body, soul, and spirit. There are over 500 Scripture verses on plants and essential oils and 422 verses on joy so you can see these are keys for your health. You were never meant to live in ordinary health or ordinary emotions. You are created to be extraordinary and joyful. I look forward to taking this journey with you!

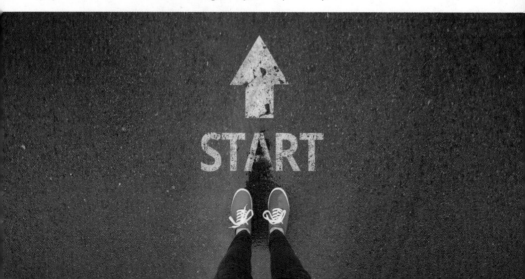

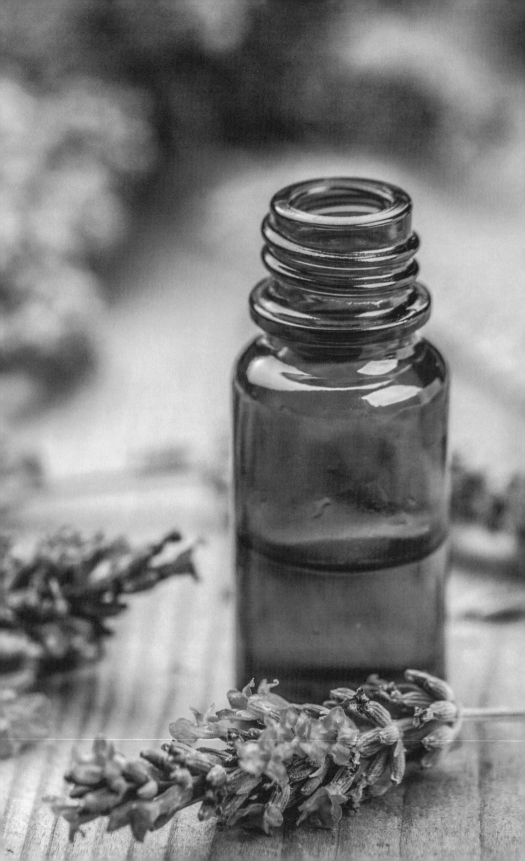

1

MY ESSENTIAL OILS STORY

F asten your seat belts; the plane is about to take off," the stewardess announced.

There was no reason to think this wouldn't be a normal flight, just like the hundreds I'd taken before. After a much-needed vacation in Florida, my husband and I were headed back to our ranch in Arizona to settle in and prepare for the birth of our third child.

But as the plane took off and began its ascent, I suddenly experienced the most awful pain. My stomach felt like it was expanding, pushing out in all directions like a pot that's overflowing.

Something was terribly wrong.

After a nauseating flight and an hour-long drive from the Phoenix airport to our ranch, I could not wait to get into bed and put my feet up.

It was too late.

At just seven and a half months along, I was in heavy labor. Despite the doctor's assurance that it was perfectly safe to fly up until eight months of pregnancy, the cabin pressure as the plane climbed into the sky had convinced my body otherwise.

Seconds later, I was on the phone with our midwife, who began coaching me while she sped to our home. As I described my labor pains, she suddenly screamed at me that I would deliver our baby in seven to ten minutes and his lungs would not be fully developed. She planned to call for a helicopter to fly me to the nearest hospital.

Without thinking, I implored her to wait a minute before making that call. The thought of being picked up, moved, and possibly delivering my baby in a helicopter was terrifying. During that one minute, I got out of bed, fell to my knees, and looked up to heaven. I cried out, "Papa, if there is anything in this house strong enough to stop heavy labor, will you please show me what it is?"

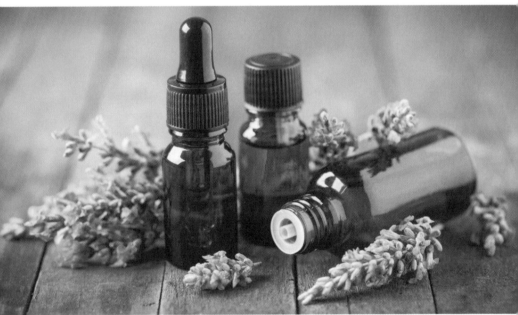

Laven[...]

Lavender to the Rescue

Instantly, three words came into my mind: *oil of lavender.* I don't know if I heard them audibly, but it seemed like they were just put into my mind as an impression. I remember looking around to see if anyone was standing there talking to me.

Lavender oil? How in the world can that help me? I was shocked. I didn't know anything about lavender oil. And in that state of mind, I did not even remember I had put Young's gift in our pantry several months earlier. But my husband ran to the pantry and came back with the bottle.

"What do I do with it?" he asked.

"I don't know," I said. "Just marinate me in it!"

We rubbed twenty drops on my stomach and few drops on the bottoms of my feet. Forty-five seconds later, the contractions stopped.

When our midwife arrived, she was frantic. She insisted we had to call for the medical helicopter. Then she paused and stared at me. "Wait a minute, what happened to you?" she asked.

"I don't know!"

She spotted the bottle of lavender oil in my hand. "What's that?"

I was still so stunned from the whole experience, I just said, "I don't know!"

She examined me and announced that the baby had dropped down so low, I had to be confined to the bed for the duration of my pregnancy—six weeks. I thought, *How is that going to happen when I have a two-year-old and a six-year-old and my husband travels all the time? She must think I'm Wonder Woman!*

Knowing the seriousness of this situation, I was determined to find a way to follow the midwife's orders. My two sisters from Denver, Jan and Jill, came to the rescue and flew down to take care of me at different times during my husband's absence. Even though I stayed in bed, lying on my side day and night, each time I got up to use the bathroom, I went right back into labor.

The first time it happened, I woke up Jan, told her I was having labor pains, and asked her to rub lavender oil on my abdomen and feet. She worked in the medical field and had never heard such a crazy idea.

Jill simply declared, "Don't you dare have this baby while I'm here!"

If reality TV shows had been popular back then, we would have had a hit comedy series on our hands.

Can I claim that the lavender oil stopped my labor? Absolutely not. However, I do know that the lavender oil, especially the fragrance, calmed me down so much that something shifted inside me and the labor just went away.

Finally, the due date arrived: November 8, 1995.

"Honey, wake up," I told our six-year-old daughter, Elizabeth. "Mommy can finally get out of bed today. Let's go for a walk." Elizabeth loved to be outdoors with me and we were horseback-riding buddies. As quickly as we could get dressed, we were out the door. She was so joyful to be outside with me. It was a glorious fall day, with birds chirping and the air smelling crisp and clean.

But within minutes, I was grabbing Elizabeth's hand, saying, "Honey, get Mommy home!" My precious little girl grabbed my hand and literally pulled me home as fast as she could. I never dreamed labor would start so quickly. Within thirty minutes, I delivered Joseph, a healthy baby boy, weighing ten pounds, three ounces. Our midwife arrived several minutes after his birth and did a beautiful job with all of my aftercare.

We were grateful to God for this safe delivery. There had been so many prayers going out for us during this time, we know He was listening.

You can imagine what was on my mind after this wild ordeal. *What in the world is lavender oil and how did it help me get through the last six weeks of my pregnancy?* But twenty-three years ago, doing research on essential oils was like trying to compete in a marathon without any running shoes. We had no computer on our ranch; our only means of communication was one giant, ugly old cell phone.

The Swiss Army Knife of Essential Oils

Nevertheless, I was relentless in my quest for answers. I learned that lavender is the Swiss Army knife of essential oils. When in doubt about which oil to use, just grab your lavender.

+ Feeling stress or pressure at work? Breathe some lavender and rub it on your shoulders.

- Having trouble getting to sleep at night? Diffuse lavender by your bedside; rub it on your feet and even on your pillow.

- Waking up in the middle of the night with restless legs? Lavender to the rescue.

- Allergies getting to you? Time to pause and breathe some lavender.

- Mild head discomfort coming on? Rub some lavender on your temples.

- Minor skin breakouts or pimples? Put a drop of lavender oil on each location.

- Want to treat yourself to a long, luxurious bath? Add about five drops of lavender oil to your bath water.

These are just a few of the hundred ways to use lavender oil.

When Joseph was old enough to talk, as I put on his pajamas at night, he would lift his feet in the air and say, "Lavender, Mommy, lavender." After marinating in that scent for six weeks in my belly, he wanted me to rub his feet with it every night.

For his sixteenth birthday, I took him to a lavender farm. For seven days, we harvested lavender together as a way of expressing gratitude to God for His provision to us in my time of need.

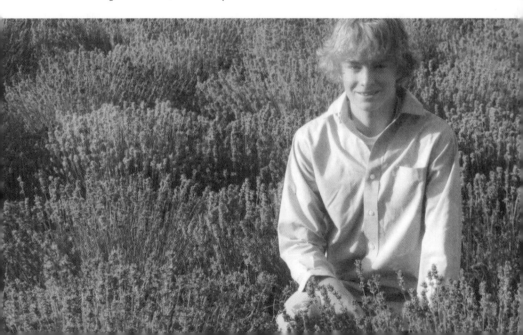

Anyone learning about essential oils today is blessed because the enormous advancements in the research, distillation, and quality of essential oils over the last twenty-five years is mind-boggling. The pathway to health with essential oils has been an arduous, daunting endeavor for the pioneers who dedicated their lives to the mission of bringing essential oils into the modern world. By the grace of God, I have been fortunate to meet and learn from some of these great pioneers. It is with a heart of thankfulness that I hope to bring this knowledge to you in a way that wakes up your heart and curiosity about the mysteries of essential oils laced throughout Scripture.

God's Provision for Our Well-Being

I believe that essential plant oils are God's extravagant provision for the well-being of our body, mind, and spirit. Just as the trees, flowers, and shrubs give us shade, color, beauty, and fragrance, their essential oils give us these same things in a highly intensified delivery system. Because it takes hundreds—and, in some cases, thousands—of pounds of plant material to create just one pound of essential oil, applying just a few drops on the body, or breathing in a few drops, can have an enormous, compounding effect.

The next time you are driving out in the country and happen to pass the most glorious, vibrant purple flowers you have ever seen, they might be wild lavender plants. If you do see them, say a little thank-you prayer. God planted them there for you and me to help us stay calm in times of stress.

During the first year I studied essential oils, the words of Scripture often seemed to jump off the page when I read a passage about trees and essential oils. There are more than 500 references to plants mentioned in the Bible and at least 200 of these refer to known aromatics. Many are described as being in pure essential oil form.

The following passage represents how the heart of God always desires to restore and heal all things for us...and let us know who's in charge.

I will turn the desert into pools of water, and the parched ground into springs. I will put in the desert the cedar and the acacia, the myrtle and

the olive. I will set junipers in the wasteland, the fir and the cypress to-
gether, so that people may see and know, may consider and understand,
that the hand of the LORD *has done this, that the Holy One of Israel*
has created it. (Isaiah 41:18–20)

This passage alone lists several trees whose essential oils support our physical and emotional health. Get ready to discover just how relevant these essential oils are for you and your family as we uncover the powerful properties of several of them in future chapters.

As a health-minded mom who looks to food as our medicine, I have discovered that there are times when food is just not enough to turn around a temporary health crisis. Our family's rallying cry is, "Oils to the rescue!"

A Terrifying Ride

When she was ten years old, Elizabeth was riding her pony through the countryside when someone on an all-terrain vehicle zoomed past her. Her terrified pony took off, dragging my daughter, whose foot was caught in a stirrup. She was tumbled, yanked, and bumped along for hundreds of yards, just like a stunt cowboy in a movie. Once her foot was finally free, I ran as fast as I could to catch up with her, scooped her up in my arms, and took her home. The minute I got her riding pants off, I gasped. A chunk of calf muscle was missing from her leg!

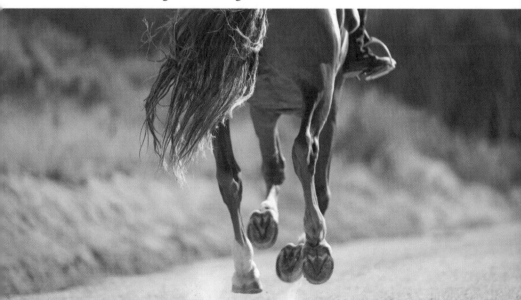

We went to the doctor's office and he ran some tests. With absolutely no emotion or compassion, he handed me a piece of paper and told me to give it to the receptionist. There was just one word on the note: *plastic*.

It did not take long before I learned that *plastic* meant plastic surgery.

"Mommy, please don't let them do surgery on me!" Elizabeth cried. "Try your oils first!"

Well, maybe a day or two might not hurt, I thought, so we went to work with my essential oils. First, I applied a blend with melaleuca (tea tree) and other essential oils to protect the wound from infection. Then I applied spikenard essential oil, as I had read several accounts of the skin-renewing qualities it contained. At night, I applied lavender and topped it off with an ointment that contained rose essential oil, which is also skin-revitalizing.

By day three, we saw so much improvement, we decided to continue on this path to see if we might actually avoid surgery. The skin continued to heal itself over several weeks until, finally, the indention had completely disappeared.

Elizabeth is now twenty-nine years old and all she has to show for that riding mishap is a tiny mark on her calf that is barely visible. Thanks to the wisdom of a child, we put God's plants to the test—and they passed.

Allow me to emphatically state that I have great respect for doctors and the sophisticated, modern-day medical field. If I had a broken bone, I wouldn't hesitate to see an orthopedic surgeon.

Natural Health Options Available

Yet I'm also aware that the education a doctor receives is limited when you consider the ever-expanding natural modalities being discovered in the world. My cousin, who's a very fine medical doctor, only received six hours of education on nutrition during six years of medical school. Good nutrition is a valuable way to avoid many diseases in the first place.

When it comes to our normal, everyday care, we need to take responsibility for our family's health. There are many situations in life when we have options. Essential oils are an option for you; however, you should

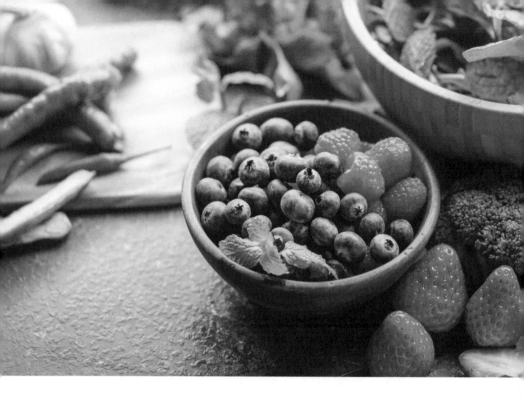

always check with your doctor before making any major health decisions. (I do hope your doctor has the compassion that everyone in the medical profession should have.)

From the time our children are born until they leave for college or work at age eighteen, we moms and dads have an awesome opportunity to nurture and nourish them on every level, including their health. Once they are out of the house and on their own, it's too late. So why not embrace the process during the at-home parenting season of life? We are only given one body on this earth and if we care for it well, it will serve us well. When childhood obesity and childhood diabetes are at epidemic stages in our nation, something is wrong. Nutrition, exercise, a positive attitude, ample sleep, and essential oils are all tools we can use every day to build a healthy body and mind.

If you are a Christ follower, I'm sure you agree we should always be learning and growing. If we truly believe God is the Great Physician, then doesn't it make sense to look for health wisdom in His Word? Scripture says, *"My people are destroyed for lack of knowledge"* (Hosea 4:6 NKJV). It does not say people will get a toothache or suffer from constipation; it says they will be destroyed.

When we look at all the wonderful believers who are suffering from debilitating illness or dying young, isn't it time to expand our understanding of Scripture in relation to health?

If I have piqued your curiosity, it's now your turn to fasten your seat belt and get ready for one of the most exciting journeys of your life—bringing the fragrance of heaven into your home, your physical body, and your heart.

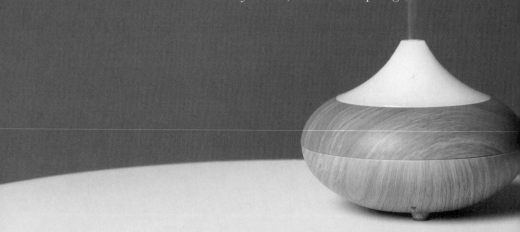

Essential oils have been a blessing to my family in so many ways! Since introducing them into my home, our immune systems are so supported, the kids haven't missed a day of school due to illness. The atmosphere created by these amazing oils is so relaxing and inviting, we have become the gathering place for the neighborhood. I highly recommend essential oils and believe that every home should have them.

—*Beverly Banks*, Colorado Springs, CO

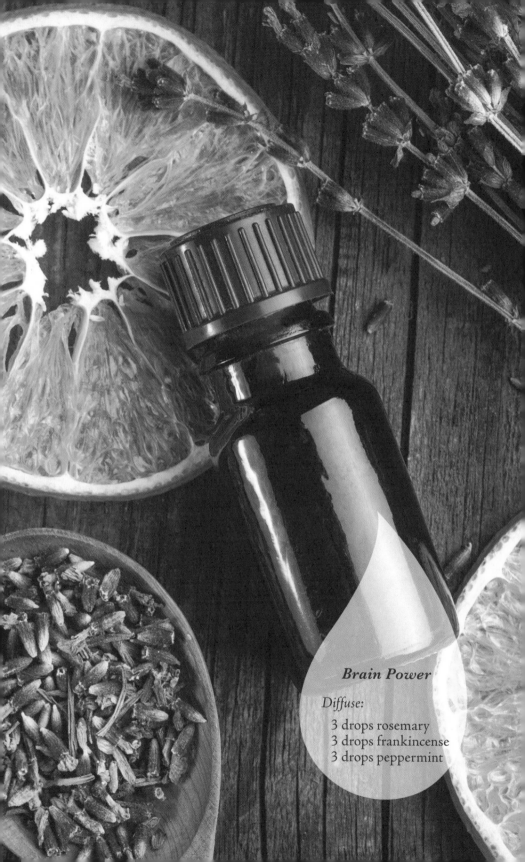

Brain Power

Diffuse:

3 drops rosemary
3 drops frankincense
3 drops peppermint

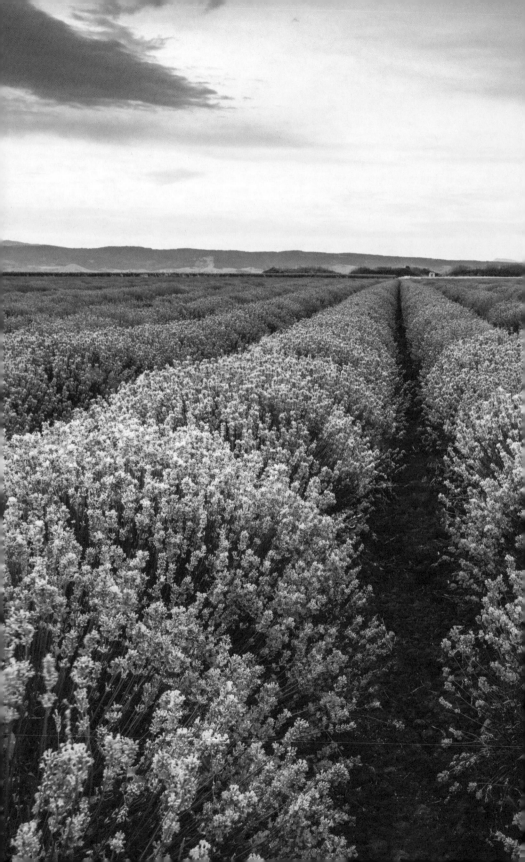

2

WHAT ARE ESSENTIAL OILS?

Close your eyes for a moment and just imagine that you are transported to the most exquisite garden you have ever seen in your life. As you walk down a garden path, what fragrances do you smell? Is it evergreen trees, spruce perhaps, luscious gardenias, exotic rose bushes, perhaps even some eucalyptus? As you breathe in these smells, can you feel your lung capacity increasing? What sounds do you hear? Perhaps the delicate whirling of hummingbirds gathering nectar, songbirds serenading you, woodpeckers drumming on tree trunks, squirrels scampering around, and babbling waterfalls and streams bringing life to every corner of the garden.

Now open your eyes. Welcome the garden of Eden! This is the lavish love the Father poured out to Adam and Eve, the same love He desires to pour on you and me. When God created Adam and Eve, He did not place them in a sterile home devoid of color, fragrance, or clean water. Instead, He placed them in a fragrant garden so they could live among rich beauty, delightful sounds, and luscious smells. This wondrous garden appeared on the third day of creation.

> The earth brought forth vegetation, plants yielding seed after their kind, and trees bearing fruit with seed in them, after their kind; and God saw that it was good. There was evening and there was morning, a third day. (Genesis 1:12–13 NASB)

The garden of Eden provided Adam and Eve with everything they needed. The trees and plants gave them wholesome, delicious food, the garden's beauty delighted their eyes, and its fragrance brought joy to their spirits. The trees, plants, and flowers offered their leaves, bark, petals, and roots for healing. These gifts, these tiny drops of "liquid gold," come straight from the heart of God's creation. They are a tool given to us so we can live in vibrant health and fulfill our destinies.

My Walk Along the Frankincense Trail

A few years ago, I had the privilege of traveling with my daughter Elizabeth to Oman in the Middle East, the only place on earth where the sacred frankincense tree grows naturally. Our guide was none other than the man who introduced me to essential oils, the late D. Gary Young. Considered the father of modern-day essential oil distillation, Young spent decades researching the ancient origins of essential oils on the Arabian Peninsula, in Egypt, and across the Mideast.

In Oman, we saw a frankincense tree that is over 700 years old and still giving its "liquid gold" sap. We traveled down the streets of Salalah, where the air is richly fragrant with frankincense. It was a wonder to behold! Salalah was a city on the Frankincense Trail, the 1,200-mile trading route connecting Oman and Yemen to the Mediterranean port in Gaza. From the fifth century B.C. through the third century A.D., the Frankincense Trail carried, at its height, 3,000 tons of precious frankincense, aromatics, and spices each year.[9]

While frankincense is used daily by people in the Middle East, the Frankincense Trail reached the West very recently. We are just now discovering the fragrant and therapeutic benefits of frankincense, so I'm thankful that it is affordable to most people today. However, when I visited Oman, I discovered that many of the ancient frankincense trees were being cut down due to the difficulty of growing and maintaining them. I hope and pray that this book will inspire frankincense growers around the world to protect these magnificent trees to ensure that our children and grandchildren will be able to experience the benefits of this amazing essential oil.

Essential oils were used in ancient Egypt, Rome, Greece, and India. According to the New World Encyclopedia, the ancient civilizations of Mesopotamia used machines to obtain essential oils from plants more than 5,000 years ago.[10]

Writing in a scholarly journal, two pharmacists noted:

"While the religious use of essential oils was recorded as early as 6000 B.C., therapeutic use of essential oils began to increase in popularity after July 1910, when [French chemist René-Maurice] Gattefossé is said to have healed burns from a laboratory explosion by quickly immersing his hands in lavender oil."[11]

During the time of Christ, essential oils were so precious, they were traded in the marketplace as if they were gold or silver coins. A king's wealth was determined in part by his possession of cinnamon oil (in India) or frankincense oil (in Israel).

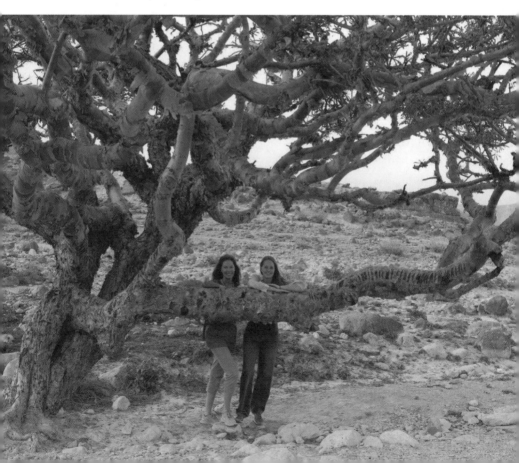

Essential Oils Explained

As we dig deeper into the power and purpose of these trees and plants, you may be wondering, *What exactly are essential oils?* If you take a leaf off of a tree or bush and tear it, you will see a drop of liquid. This is the plant's essential oil—essential because plants cannot live without this oil. If a plant is damaged, the oil comes to the rescue, heals the plant, and restores it to health. In the same way, essential oils are compatible with the human body; they help to heal it and restore it to health.

Oils Contain Powerful Chemicals

Essential oils contain several powerful, natural chemical constituents. Three of the most important ones are:

- Phenylpropanoids, which cleanse the cell's receptor sites. Receptor sites are instrumental in getting important information to our cells.

- Sesquiterpenes, which help to erase incorrect information in the cellular memory.

- Monoterpenes, which help to restore God's original image into the DNA.

So these drops of "liquid gold" help us to return to the image of God in which we were created. The best part is that when used correctly, there are no negative side effects with essential oils because they are part of the plant kingdom given to us on the third day of creation. Essential oils strengthen our bodies, support our health, and give us the boost we need to heal.

Traditional drugs focus on the symptom. When a drug is created to kill bacteria, some members of that bacteria colony may mutate so that they become resistant to the drug. "Misuse and overuse of these drugs… have contributed to a phenomenon known as antibiotic resistance," notes the U.S. Food and Drug Administration. "This resistance develops when potentially harmful bacteria change in a way that reduces or eliminates the effectiveness of antibiotics."[12]

Get enough of these resistant bacteria together and you may have an outbreak of a disease like Methicillin-resistant Staphylococcus aureus

(MRSA). Many essential oils strengthen the body's defenses so that it can fight off or kill the bacteria.

Distilling Essential Oils

The process of extracting oil from plants to create an essential oil cannot be learned overnight. The art of distillation requires years of study, a keen understanding of plants, and relentless dedication. Every plant, flower, shrub, and tree is unique. Harvesting them for their oil, distilling the raw materials, and controlling the temperature demands precision and care. I like to compare those who manufacture essential oils to musicians in a symphony orchestra.

For example, think about one of the most fragrant flowers on earth: the rose. Imagine two semitrucks driving down the highway, carrying 5,000 pounds of rose petals. These beautiful petals arrive at the distillery, where they are placed in large, stainless-steel containers known as distillers. The petals are then distilled at a very low temperature and over a long period of time to preserve the delicate healing properties of rose oil. I recommend therapeutic-grade essential oils, which have nothing added during the distillation process—no fillers, no chemicals, nothing.

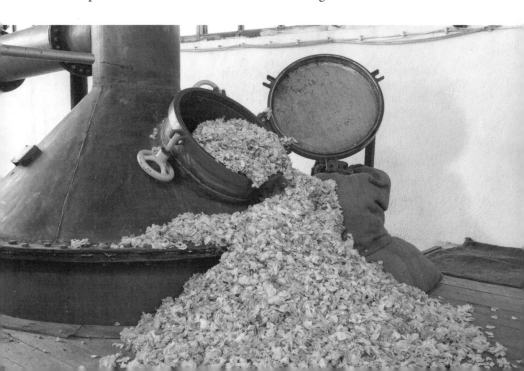

Once the rose petals have gone through this process, the finished product weighs one pound. Yes, you read that correctly: it takes 5,000 pounds of rose petals to make one pound of glorious rose essential oil. Essential oils are super-concentrated, so just a few drops can have a significant impact on your well-being.

Different techniques are used to harvest the raw plant material that's used to create essential oils. For instance, frankincense oil is extracted from the Boswellia tree by cutting into the bark. This cut releases a thick, creamy sap, which is collected and distilled. Fortunately, the tree heals itself, so this process can be repeated hundreds of times over the life of a tree, allowing its sap to benefit many people for years.

Let Quality Be Your Guide

Throughout this book, I use the term *therapeutic-grade essential oils* to distinguish the highest-quality oils from others. There is no industry standard for grading essential oils, but there are other ways to distinguish quality products. The highest quality essential oil is:

+ Distilled from plants grown without the harmful use of pesticides and herbicides
+ Distilled at a low temperature for a long period of time to preserve the source plant's delicate therapeutic characteristics
+ One hundred percent essential oil, with no adulterants, synthetic chemicals, fragrances, colorants, or additives
+ Labeled GRAS (Generally Regarded as Safe) if it is a supplement-grade essential oil

If a product is labeled "pure," that is not necessarily an indication of quality. By law, an essential oil labeled "pure" is only required to be 10 percent essential oil. The remaining 90 percent of the product can be synthetic fragrance, water, or other ingredients.

God's Loving Gifts to Us

Are you starting to see how generous and loving God was when He gave us so many different trees and plants on the third day of creation?

As a health and wellness coach, I work with over two hundred essential oils. However, I can show the average family how to improve their daily health by just starting with a few essential oils.

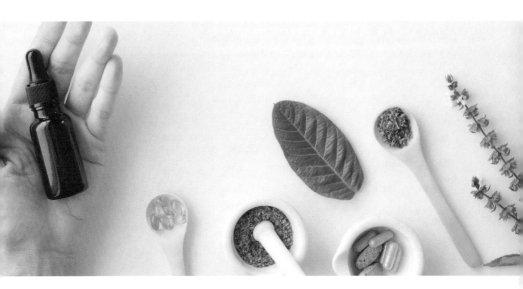

Ways to Use Essential Oils

There are three primary ways we use essential oils and a few other secondary ways that they can benefit our health and wellbeing. (See chapter 6, Supporting Each System of the Body, for specific uses of different essential oils.)

1. Topical

As your body's largest organ, your skin is a magnificent delivery system for essential oils. Think of it as a living, breathing organism. If I take some olive oil and pour it into your hand, unless you move or dump it out, that oil will still be sitting in your hand twenty minutes from now. Yet if I take some essential oil such as frankincense and pour it into your hand, the oil will dissipate in just a few minutes. The essential oil molecules are so tiny, they easily penetrate your skin. Thus, your body can receive the benefits of the oil without it having to go through the digestive system or liver. God made your skin to be the most amazing delivery system ever.

Unlike cold-pressed vegetable oils such as olive oil or coconut oil, essential oils are volatile liquids that dissipate rapidly. When placed on the bottoms of your feet or along your spine, essential oil reaches every system of your body through your nerve endings. Your nerves act like the stems and veins of a plant, transporting the oil to the area of your body that needs it.

Common Sense Precautions

Some essential oils, such as oregano, thyme, and cinnamon bark, are high in phenols and may need to be diluted because they can be caustic to the skin. A good way to test an essential oil is by placing a drop on your arm. If it stings a little bit, you will want to dilute it. To dilute an essential oil, simply take a few drops of olive oil in the palm of your hand and add a few drops of essential oil before applying. You could also use another oil such as almond, coconut, grape seed, or sesame seed for dilution purposes.

Never put essential oils in your eyes, ears, or private areas. If you accidently rub your eyes with oil on them, put a few drops of olive oil—not water—in your eyes and blink.

Your great-grandmother might have gone out to her garden or into a nearby field or woods to pick herbs for a poultice to rub on the chest of a sick child suffering from congestion. You have a much easier means of improving your health at your disposal. All you need to do is open a bottle of essential oil, place a few drops in your hands, and rub it on the area of your body in need of healing. It's that simple.

Perhaps you have sore knees after a run or a workout. Rub essential oil on your knees and you should experience relief rather quickly. If you're in a lot of pain, you may need to try additional applications.

Suppose your chest feels a little tight after walking the dog or running errands on a cold, blustery day. Rub a few drops of essential oils right on your chest and, if need be, over your lungs. The pores of your skin will capture the oils and transport these soothing drops to the area where you need them.

Or, using another example, maybe you've had a very long, difficult day at work and you're feeling upset, angry, or agitated. As the Stevie Wonder song goes, "Don't You Worry 'bout a Thing."[13] Pour about ten drops of lavender oil in the bottom of your bathtub, fill it with warm water, and soak in the tub for at least twenty minutes. This is just the ticket for frayed nerves.

If you're not sure where the essential oils should be rubbed on your body, just place them on your feet or have someone rub them down your spine. Your nerve endings will capture the oil and transport it throughout your entire body in about twenty minutes.

You may be thinking, *Hmm, really?* If you have doubts, try this test: take a fresh clove of garlic (not minced garlic sold in a jar), chop it into tiny pieces, and rub it on the bottoms of your feet. In twenty minutes, ask a family member if you have garlic breath. Be prepared for them to wave you away. This test works every time and illustrates the power of the nerve endings in your feet to transport essential oils throughout your body.

2. Inhalation

We have five senses: sight, smell, hearing, taste, and touch. Yet until very recently, little attention was paid to the importance of our sense of smell. Today, modern science is flooding us with exciting research on the amazing power that this sense has on our emotions.

In fact, some leading international researchers have gathered in Stockholm, Sweden, to investigate how the mind processes olfaction—the sense of smell. This six-year research program, entitled Our Unique Sense

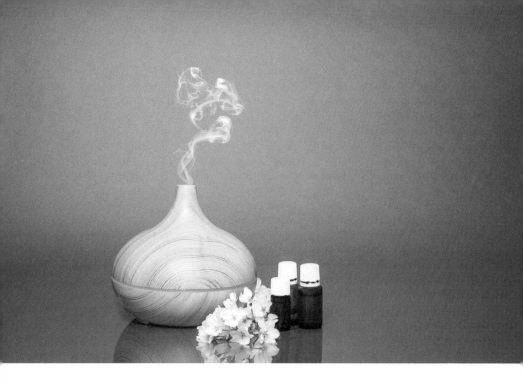

of Smell (OUSOS), is funded by a $3.7 million grant from the Swedish Foundation for Humanities and Social Sciences.[14] It will conclude in February 2021.

One of the most surprising things I've learned about essential oils is the powerful way they help to support positive emotions and release negative emotions. When you breathe in an essential oil, its properties travel from your nostrils to the olfactory bulb—an area of the forebrain that detects odors—to the amygdala region of your brain in just three seconds. Located in the frontal portion of the temporal lobe, the amygdala is the seat of our emotions; every emotion and memory from our life is recorded here. It's essential to our ability to feel certain emotions and perceive them in other people.

Unless we cannot hear, we know that most of our brain responds to sound. However, the amygdala only responds to scent. Depending upon which essential oil you breathe, as soon as the scent molecules reach the amygdala, the brain becomes a communication system within the body and tells it what to do.

For example, when you are stressed out and feeling overwhelmed, as soon as you begin breathing lavender essential oil, your brain speaks to your body and tells it to let go of the stress. Suddenly, your shoulders relax and your feeling of being overwhelmed is diminished.

This information has life-changing possibilities for you and your family.

Anointed and Healed

A few years ago, I had the privilege of being part of a ministry trip to Bali, Indonesia. I was invited to give a short talk on "Healing Emotions with Essential Oils." Immediately afterward, a beautiful young woman came up to me and asked if I would anoint her with oil. I knew nothing about her life, so I anointed her head with frankincense, put several drops of this oil in her hands, and invited her to breathe it in.

Shortly after I began to pray for her, she started to weep…and continued to do so for about forty-five minutes as I prayed and tried to comfort her. Then she told me her story. She was born in China and at that time, it was illegal to have more than one child. In an attempt to hide her pregnancy, her mother went to live with a relative when she was six months' along—and then gave this woman away on the day of her birth. This young woman had never even seen her mother's face.

As the prayers went forth to heaven that day, this precious woman had a full vision of her mother. She saw her mother's face and watched her pace back and forth, holding her swollen belly protectively. The woman told me that all of her life, she had been walking around holding her own stomach and never knew why. She said, "Teri, I now know that my mother loved me and she was trying to protect me. And now, I no longer have to walk around this way."

This was a joyful moment for all who were present and a great example of God's lavish love and the tools of prayer and anointing that He gave us for healing.

The best way to get to know an essential oil is by pouring a couple of drops in your hands, rubbing your hands together, cupping them over your nose, and breathing deeply. If you are breathing peppermint oil, you will be amazed at how it wakes you up, opens your sinuses, energizes you almost instantly, and makes you feel more alive. Breathing lavender oil will have the exact opposite effect; you will notice your shoulders relax, your tension release, and a calmness come over you. In fact, you may suddenly want to take a nap!

Each plant that God gave us is 100 percent unique and designed to address particular health needs throughout our lifetime.

One of my favorite ways to inhale essential oils is with the use of a cold air or cold-water diffuser. There are so many benefits of diffusing, the first being that the smell creates a special atmosphere in your home. When my three children were young, they often came running into the house after playing outside and declared, "Mommy, turn on the joy, turn on the joy!" Without even knowing why, they were begging me to turn on the diffuser and related the smells coming out of it as joyful.

The second benefit is that essential oils can cleanse and purify the air in your home. Imagine having a group of people over and a few have the sniffles. By diffusing frankincense and tangerine essential oil into the air, not only will your home smell lovely, but you will be actively supporting the well-being of your guests.

Third, pet owners absolutely love the effects of diffusing oils to calm and relieve the anxiety of a hyper or nervous pet. Make sure to place your diffuser into an area that your pet cannot reach and add five to ten drops of lavender.

3. Internal

The use of essential oils internally is highly effective, but it must be accompanied by knowledge and understanding of how to safely ingest them, which oils can be consumed, and which cannot.

Here are some important points to keep in mind:

+   Always consult with your doctor before using essential oils internally.

+   Only ingest those essential oils that have been certified for internal use and only in small amounts. The vast majority of essential oils sold in grocery and health food stores are labeled "Not for Internal Use." This is an indication that the oil is not supplement-grade.

One of my favorite ways to use essential oils internally is to add citrus oils to my drinking water. In the morning, I take a glass pitcher and add a few drops of citrus oil—such as lemon, orange, tangerine, grapefruit, or lime—and a drop of peppermint oil. I fill the pitcher with pure, filtered water and place it on my counter or in the refrigerator and drink it all day long. Water used to be such a boring beverage, but no more. It's now an exciting adventure as every day, the water tastes subtly different and each glass is so satisfying.

If you are looking for something to curb your appetite, peppermint is your friend. The properties in peppermint oil help to create a feeling of being satiated. Try adding a drop to a glass of water or a single drop on your tongue. As a bonus, you'll have fresh, minty breath.

Supplement-grade oils are the best for flavoring food. Almost every herb that you might use for cooking also comes in essential oil form, including basil, oregano, thyme, and marjoram. Because an essential oil has never been dried like an herb, it is more powerful, so a tiny bit goes a long way, making them very affordable. I usually start by dipping a toothpick

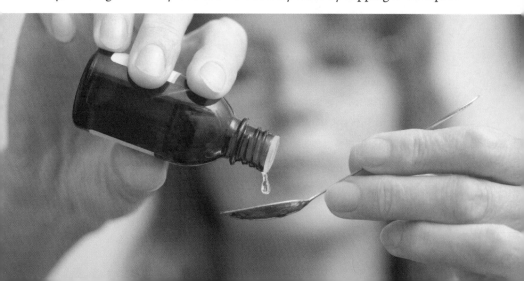

into my essential oil bottle and then stirring the toothpick into whatever I'm cooking, such as chili or spaghetti sauce. You can always add more, but once in the recipe, you can never take it away.

If you feel like your favorite recipes are starting to taste rather humdrum, it's time to try adding some essential oils. Salad dressings come alive with tanginess. Desserts become layers of surprising flavors with just a drop or two of peppermint, lemon, lime, tangerine, nutmeg, or cinnamon essential oils.

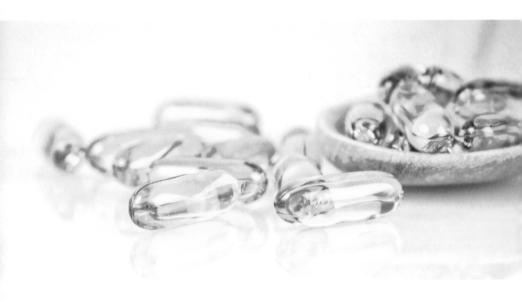

Another internal application of oils consists of placing a few drops of an essential oil in an empty gel capsule and then filling up the capsule with almond milk or olive oil. Our family avoided untold numbers of doctor visits simply by being proactive at the onset of sniffles and using the essential oils that support a healthy immune system response. Rather than the symptoms turning into a full-fledged cold, we like to take a blend of oils internally that encourage the body's natural defenses to kick into high gear. This includes cinnamon, clove, lemon, eucalyptus, and rosemary.

There are many ways to incorporate essential oils into your daily life.

Over the years of raising three animal-loving children, we have owned dogs, cats, turtles, rabbits, ponies, and horses. We've discovered that animals can also benefit from essential oils. You might say our animals have been a bit of an experiment when it comes to oils. The results have been exceptional.

We had a hunter/jumper thoroughbred horse who suffered from over-the-top anxiety. Imagine our surprise when we applied lavender oil to the frog of his hoofs (i.e., the V-shaped area that acts as a shock absorber) and he suddenly became Mr. Calm and Confident!

That same lavender went on our dog's paws, shifting him from an uncontrollable puppy to an easygoing, lovable lapdog. You can find some helpful reference books in many bookstores or in the library on how to safely and effectively use essential oils on your pets.

Essential oils weave a complex, rich tapestry of life-giving molecules that provide support for our physical, emotional, mental, and spiritual health. They are God's provision for all aspects of our life and as they become an everyday part of your life, you may start to wonder how in the world you ever got along without them.

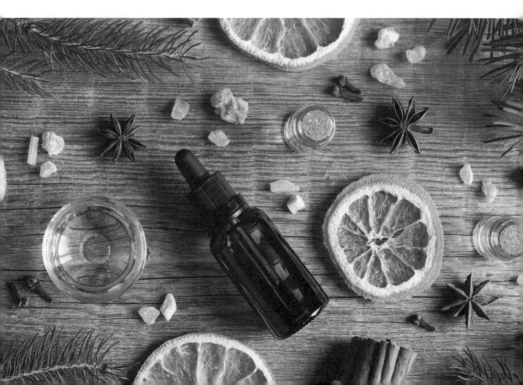

LET YOUR EYES LOOK STRAIGHT AHEAD; FIX YOUR GAZE DIRECTLY BEFORE YOU.

—PROVERBS 4:25

Focus

Diffuse:

 3 drops grapefruit
 3 drops basil
 3 drops cedarwood

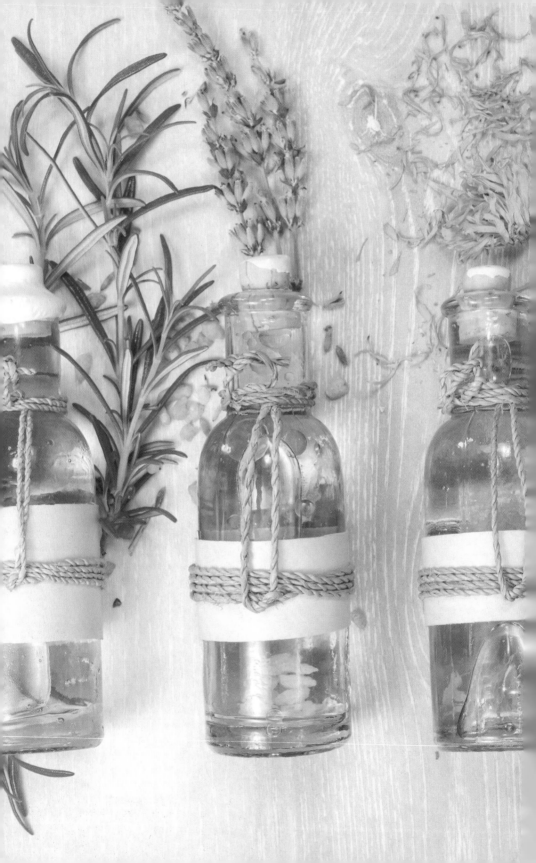

3

A CLOSER LOOK AT JAMES 5:14

One of the greatest personal revelations I received years ago was God's instruction to anoint others with essential oils, not olive oil, before prayer. This is one of God's provisions for the healing of body, mind, emotions, and spirit. It's right in the Bible and it's one of my favorite passages in Scripture:

> *Is any sick among you? Let him call for the elders of the church; and let them pray over him, anointing him with oil in the name of the Lord.*
> (James 5:14 KJV)

Yes, God really does instruct us to anoint the sick with oils when we pray.

You may wonder, *But why can't a person just get healed through prayer?* Yes, a person can absolutely get healed just through prayer; we see it all of the time. I have also frequently witnessed people receiving healing with a combination of prayer and precious oils. Remember, God is very creative and can heal any way He desires.

To more fully understand this passage in James, let's examine the word "anoint." According to *Vine's Expository Dictionary*, "The Hebrew word for 'anoint' is *masach*, which means to smear, spread, or massage. In some cases, it means to pour oil all over the head and body."

That's no small amount of oil! If "precious oil" was used, that would be costly indeed. Such oil was part of a king's treasury. Showing off his wealth to his royal visitors from Babylon, King Hezekiah *"hearkened unto them, and showed them all the house of his precious things, the silver, and the gold, and the spices, and the precious oil, and the house of his armor, and all that was found in his treasures"* (2 Kings 20:13 ASV).

Author David Stewart, a retired Methodist minister and former science professor, has researched essential oils mentioned in the Bible and their healing applications. He writes, "The word 'precious' was never applied to olive oil alone, but always indicated the use of essential oils such as cassia, hyssop, and frankincense."[15]

Different Types of Healing

Since God instructs us to pray and anoint with precious oils, there must be a reason. Sorting through a couple of Greek words here, I think you will find the answer. In the New Testament, the Greek word *iaomai* is defined as instantaneous healing. *Iaomai* is mentioned thirty times in the Gospels and it refers to those times when God heals someone immediately. We see many examples of this laced throughout Scripture.

Another important Greek word in the New Testament is *therapeuo*, the word from which therapy is derived. *Therapeuo* means to "serve" or "attend to" as in "to heal gradually over time with care and nursing." This may include self-administered care such as exercise, rest, change of attitude and diet, and daily anointing with essential oils. *Therapeuo* is mentioned forty times in the New Testament. This healing takes natural law into account and the opportunity we have to honor our bodies and treat them as the temples God designed them to be. I truly believe it is always our Creator's delight to heal us.

Both types of healing are miraculous and demonstrate the love and compassion of our Lord.

Since *therapeuo* or therapeutic healing is mentioned ten more times than *iaomai* or instantaneous healing in the New Testament, we should take note of this and examine all of the elements involved in *therapeuo* healing. It's time to lift our hearts and minds to our Creator and give sincere consideration into making a greater effort toward a healthier lifestyle, especially if we don't feel well or know we aren't in the best of health.

John 10:10 says, "*The thief comes only to steal and kill and destroy; I came that they may have life, and have it abundantly*" (NASB).

The enemy of your soul will try to destroy your health, your marriage, your career, your finances, and your joy. But Jesus came that we might have life and have it more abundantly—all of it, including our health.

Once we are healed, we can honor God by taking care of our bodies and turning away from the things that harmed us in the first place, such as negative thought patterns or an unhealthy lifestyle. If we were all vibrant, energetic, and clear-minded—wow! Wouldn't that be great? But that's not the case, so we need to change how we think about what we put into our bodies.

You Can Still Have Chocolate, But...

Does this mean we can never enjoy a piece of chocolate? Of course not! Even if we eat well just 80 percent of the time, our livers can probably handle the not-so-good choices we make the other 20 percent of the time. However, if you look at what people put into their grocery carts, often it's

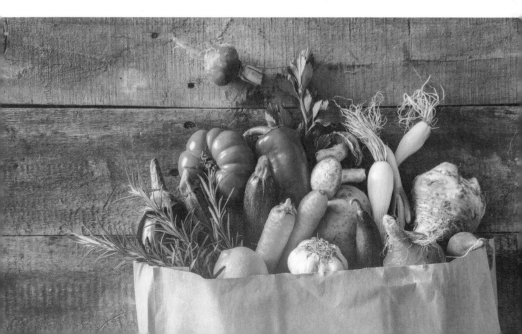

more like 20 percent healthy, nutritious foods and 80 "junk" or unwholesome foods like potato chips, sodas, sugary cereals, cookies, and the like. Our livers simply cannot handle this kind of stress.

Yet the very Spirit of God makes His home inside us, as this thrilling account from Scripture relates:

> *Do you not know that your body is a temple of the Holy Spirit within you, whom you have from God? You are not your own, for you were bought with a price. So glorify God in your body.*
> (1 Corinthians 6:19–20 ESV)

This thought is just riveting to me and I hope it inspires you, too.

Think of your body as a beautiful home awaiting a treasured guest, the Holy Spirit of God. If your home is full of love, peace, grace, light, and health, the Spirit arrives and gently, happily settles in to His glorious home. But what if the Spirit knocks on the door of your home and as you open it, He discerns sickness, spoiled food, negative thoughts, judgment, and mockery? Do you think He would want to stay?

Every day is a new day that offers us the opportunity to become better. Thinking life-giving thoughts, choosing life-giving words, and eating life-giving foods and substances produce a life of abundance.

You may be thinking, *But hasn't the church been using olive oil for years to anoint people?* Yes, that's true. But God gave us the recipe for a holy anointing oil thousands of years ago.

> *The LORD said to Moses, "Take the following fine spices: 500 shekels of liquid **myrrh**, half as much (that is, 250 shekels) of fragrant **cinnamon**, 250 shekels of fragrant **calamus**, 500 shekels of **cassia**—all according to the sanctuary shekel—and a hin of olive oil. Make these into a sacred anointing oil, a fragrant blend, the work of a perfumer. It will be the sacred anointing oil."*
> (Exodus 30:22–25)

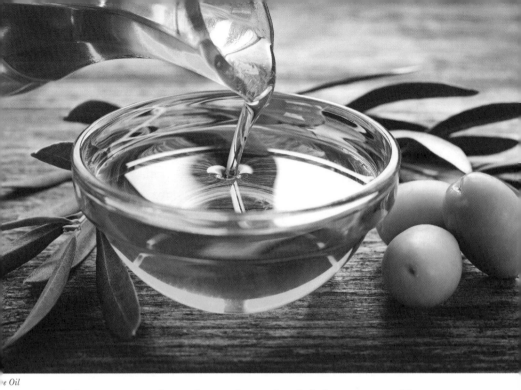

Other versions refer to the resulting oil as "*a holy anointing oil.*"

Earlier, "*the LORD SAID TO MOSES, 'Tell the Israelites to bring me an offering. ...olive oil for the light;* **spices for the anointing oil** *and for the* **fragrant incense**'" (Exodus 25:1–2, 6).

The spices mentioned here refer to cinnamon, clove, cassia (which is similar to cinnamon), frankincense, and all of the sweet incense that comes from fragrant plants. God put something extra special in His fragrant plants that can be used to help the body heal.

The Significance of James 5:14

Several years ago, as I was contemplating the significance of James 5:14, I just blurted out, "Papa, can you please give me a picture of the real meaning of James 5:14?" The image that God placed in my mind was that of a sick man lying in bed. His wife called the elders of the church, who came and gathered at his bedside. Soon, they were praying and anointing his feet, his spine, and his head with essential oils. I saw them apply the oils a second time, followed by more prayer, and then a third time, with more prayers lifted up to God for the man's healing. Suddenly, the man sat up, got out of bed, and started to walk.

Wow, I thought, *this is exciting!* The man was not confined to bed for a week or a month; he just got up and walked around. Why? Because there is power in prayer and there are healing properties in the plants God gave us on the third day of creation to help the body heal itself.

Just because I saw a mental image of the elders anointing the man three times does not mean that *you* must anoint someone three times. Remember, Jesus Himself healed people differently each time. As we become more and more sensitive to the Holy Spirit, we will be shown what to do in each situation.

You *Are Qualified to Pray*

So, who are the church elders today? If you are a man or woman of faith and put your trust in the true and living God, *you* are qualified to pray for people. Don't be shy. Prayer and anointing with oils are meant to be a normal, everyday occurrence in families, like brushing your teeth or making your bed.

When a quarterback throws a football, he throws it like he means it. When you pray, pray like you mean it! God loves it when our prayers are passionate. He already knows what's on your mind; He desires to know what's in your heart.

One of the greatest answers I ever received in prayer happened when I was walking along a beach in Florida while crying my eyes out in desperation for the Lord to hear and answer an ongoing prayer of mine. That day, I prayed like I meant it and He answered like He meant it. Very few things in life get settled on an intellectual level; just about everything gets settled on an emotional level, in our hearts.

Anointing in the Bible

The instruction in James 5:14 to pray and anoint with oils is not merely symbolic, as some types of prayer ritual may be. Every single tree, flower, shrub, herb, and plant in the world has distinct qualities that our bodies can use to restore health to us. Once you open the door of your heart to the concept of anointing, you will be thrilled to learn that it is absolutely everywhere in Scripture.

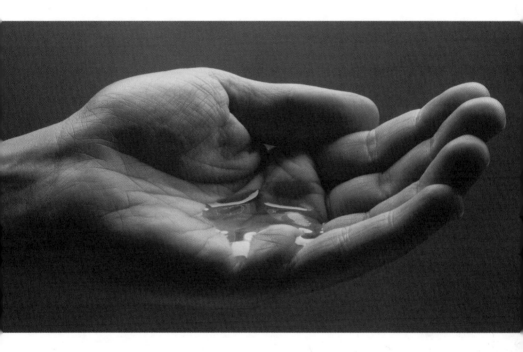

The Anointing of Aaron

One example I love is how God told Moses to anoint Aaron to set him apart and prepare him for priestly service to the Lord:

After you put these clothes on your brother Aaron and his sons, anoint and ordain them. Consecrate them so they may serve me as priests.
(Exodus 28:41)

King David sang of this anointing thus: *"It is like the precious ointment upon the head, that ran down upon the beard, even Aaron's beard: that went down to the skirts of his garments"* (Psalm 133:2 kjv).

Can you imagine being anointed with so much oil that it just runs all over you and all over your clothes? Not only that, but this was a family affair. Aaron and his sons were all anointed and set apart for the service of the Lord, through the anointing of oil in a most dramatic way. I believe the fragrance created an atmosphere absolutely thick with joy on that day. Remember, God is extravagant! So when you use your oils, choose to be extravagant with yourself. God is watching as you breathe in the life-giving fragrances.

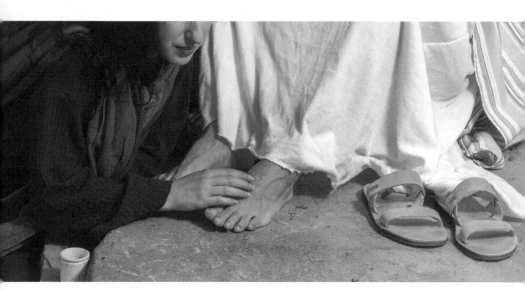

The Anointing of Jesus

Speaking of extravagance, all four gospels provide accounts of a woman anointing Jesus with an expensive perfume or ointment. Two gospels say a woman poured the perfume on the Lord's head (see Matthew 26:6–13; Mark 14:3–9), while the other two say a woman anointed Jesus's feet (Luke 7:36–50; John 12:1–8).

John writes, *"Mary took about a pint of pure nard, an expensive perfume; she poured it on Jesus' feet and wiped his feet with her hair. And the house was filled with the fragrance of the perfume"* (John 12:3).

Nard, also known as spikenard, is an aromatic, amber-colored essential oil derived from a flowering plant in the valerian family that grows in the Himalayas of Nepal, China, and India. The amount of spikenard oil that Mary poured on Jesus was worth about three hundred days' wages.

This oil is also mentioned in the Song of Songs, with the Shulamite, the country maiden, saying, *"While the king sat at his table, my spikenard sent forth its fragrance"* (Song of Solomon 1:12 ASV).

The Anointing of David

> *So Samuel took the horn of oil and anointed him in the presence of his brothers, and from that day on the spirit of the LORD came powerfully upon David.* (1 Samuel 16:13)

Anointing for Hospitality

According to Jewish tradition, it was an act of hospitality to wash and anoint the feet of a visitor who had traveled a long distance to come to your home. Naturally, the scent of the oils would cover up any unpleasant smell associated with travelling in the heat and the dust.

Yet, the best part to keep in mind is that it created a pleasant and welcoming atmosphere the moment your guest arrived. Today, many people use essential oil diffusers in their homes to create the same welcoming scent. As an added benefit, certain citrus oils—such as lemon, orange, tangerine, and grapefruit—are known to be emotionally uplifting!

Holy Anointing Oil in Exodus

Taking a closer look at God's recipe for holy anointing oil that He gave to Moses in Exodus 30:23–24, we see that this oil was to be used by the priests to anoint and cleanse themselves and everything in the temple. It was made from myrrh, cassia, cinnamon, calamus, and olive oil. It's estimated that this recipe yielded almost six gallons of anointing oil that would be valued at around $150,000 today. So God's goal in giving Moses this recipe was not for some mere symbolic act. The oil was a lavish extravagance! God lavishes His love, His fragrance, and His joy on those who will receive it.

When we examine the unique properties of these four essential oils, we can see why they were used to make the holy anointing oil and why you could benefit from them today.

Myrrh

The scent of myrrh is an earthy, grounding fragrance, promoting feelings of peace and relaxation. Myrrh essential oil supports a healthy immune system, reduces the look of fine lines, wrinkles, and blemishes, and promotes skin healing. Some scientific studies suggest that myrrh may protect against gum disease and inflammation; it may also have antibacterial properties for dental patients undergoing root canals.[16]

Cassia

Cassia's fragrance is similar to cinnamon's, but slightly mellower. The scent of cassia lifts the spirits and infuses the body with a gentle energy. It also supports the immune system, builds the body's natural defenses, and supports healthy digestion.

Cinna

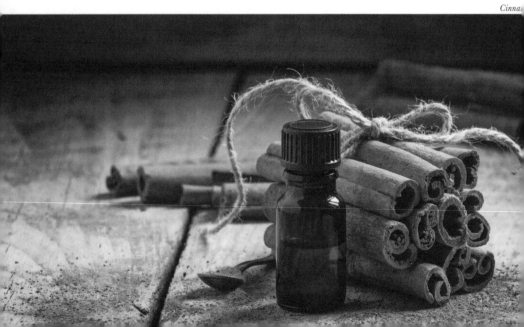

Cinnamon

Cinnamon supports the cardiovascular and digestive systems; it may also support healthy blood sugar levels. A study in *Current Neurology and Neuroscience Reports* found that cinnamon essential oil was effective in significantly reducing a type of bacteria linked to the development of dental cavities.[17]

The sweet and spicy fragrance of cinnamon is known to relax the senses and deepen awareness for our surroundings.

Calamus

Calamus, also known as sweet flag, is believed to have numerous medicinal properties, including serving as a muscle relaxant, central nervous system depressant, anticonvulsant, analgesic, and sedative.

The plant "seems to have originated in India or Arabia but is now found in many places throughout the world," wrote essential oils researcher Gary Young. "Native Americans used calamus as a medicine and a stimulant, but low doses are also believed to be calming and to induce sleep. The Penobscot people have a tradition that it saved their people from a serious illness."[18]

mus

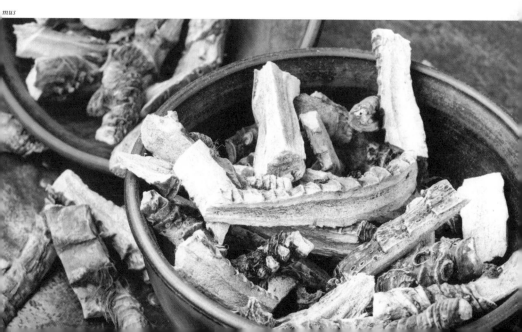

God's Special Perfume

God's directions for the creation of holy anointing oil was not the only recipe that the Lord gave to Moses. He also provided the formula for His very own exquisite perfume. That's right—our Creator loves scent!

And the Lord *said to Moses: "Take sweet spices,* **stacte** *and* **onycha** *and* **galbanum,** *and pure* **frankincense** *with these sweet spices; there shall be equal amounts of each. You shall make of these an incense, a compound according to the art of the perfumer, salted, pure, and holy.... You shall not make any for yourselves, according to its composition. It shall be to you holy for the* Lord."

(Exodus 30:34–35, 37 nkjv)

The Scripture says this formula is not to be copied or made for personal use, as it is holy to the Lord for His pleasure.

Imagine this: every time you turn on a diffuser in your home, your office, or even in a church, and spread the fragrance of an essential oil such as frankincense into the air, your heavenly Father is enjoying it right along with you. I can't help but smile from ear to ear when I think of this.

We have already looked at stacte, which is another biblical word for myrrh. Here are the significant properties of the other three spices in God's special perfume:

Onycha

The deep, vanilla-like scent of onycha is known to heighten your spiritual awareness and move you into a state of relaxation. This scent can be helpful in releasing past emotions.

Onycha has been known to support healthy digestion and maintaining a healthy blood sugar level.

Due to its powerful antiseptic properties, onycha was once used throughout the world to fumigate hospitals.[19] Burning this oil in the Lord's temple would essentially fumigate it and keep the air free from germs.

Galbanum

Galbanum is used in many cosmetics and skin care products because of its ability to beautify and heal the skin.[20] Those with mature skin can use galbanum in conjunction with sandalwood to reduce the look of fine lines and wrinkles.[21]

The scent of galbanum is reminiscent of bell peppers. It's been known to help with deep, negative emotions such as anger and frustration.[22]

Frankincense

Frankincense has a deep woody aroma with a hint of lemon. Its scent has been known to expand consciousness and deepen prayer.

Frankincense is a powerful, effective essential oil with therapeutic benefits for the skin and hair, respiratory system, and immune system. Frankincense eases the clearing of nasal passages and lungs due to colds and coughs.

When diffused, frankincense eliminates airborne bacteria and fungi, making for a healthy indoor environment for your family.[23]

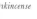
nkincense

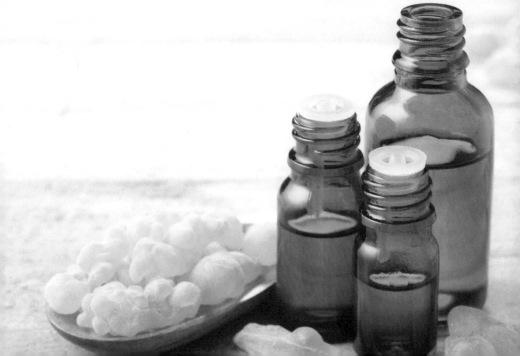

Some studies also show that frankincense increases mobility for those with osteoarthritis.[24]

God Lavishes Love on My Father

In 1981, my parents and my sister, Kathy, were traveling during a horrible Iowa snowstorm when their car was struck by a drunk driver. My dear mother and beautiful sister were killed instantly; Dad suffered multiple, life-threatening injuries. It took a long time for Dad to recover physically, and for my three remaining siblings and me to recover emotionally.

Years later, the injuries that Dad incurred in that tragic accident caused him to have a major stroke. It left him confined to a bed at the Iowa Veterans Home in Marshalltown, Iowa, completely paralyzed on one side of his body and unable to walk, talk, or eat.

Dad had been in the home for ten years when I had my miraculous lavender experience during my pregnancy with Joseph. It wasn't long afterward that I wondered if essential oils could work in a preventive or protective way for my Dad, who often suffered from colds or the flu.

Frankincense and M

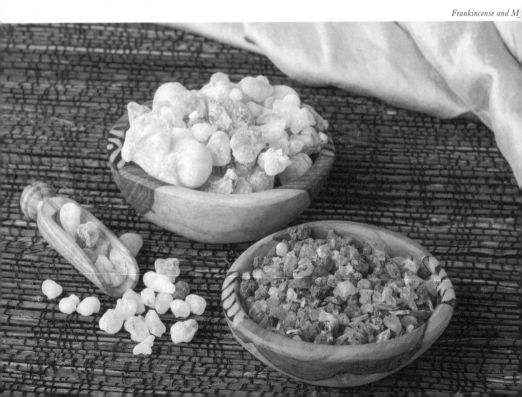

If It's Good Enough for Jesus...

I called the Iowa Veterans Home and ran my idea past them. After several months, they gave permission for Dad to be anointed with essential oil down his spine once a day. When his nurse called with the good news, she asked me which oils I would like her to use. Because I was so new to essential oils and really knew nothing about choosing them for a specific goal, I blurted out, "Frankincense and myrrh." I just figured that if they were good enough for Christ, they must certainly be good for my Dad.

I sent these powerful essential oils to the nurse with the understanding that she would only have time to place three or four drops of each oil down his spine once a day after his shower. While this is a very mild application, I figured this was surely better than nothing.

After thirty days, Dad's nurse called and told me that a very bad flu virus was going around the Iowa Veterans Home and most of the doctors had gone home sick. Then she said, "Teri, I do not know what it is about these oils, but your Dad has not had even the slightest sniffle." Since she was afraid she might get the flu as well, she said, "Every time I start to feel sick, I just run into your Dad's room and begin to sniff the frankincense and I immediately get over it!"

This news made my heart sing. It had been my hope to keep Dad more comfortable and avoid unnecessary illness. I was so happy!

His Eyes Twinkle as He Lifts an Arm

Sixty more days went by and then came another call from Dad's nurse. Her voice was trembling and I feared the worst.

"Teri," she said, "you know I have been your Dad's nurse for ten years and you know that he has never moved a muscle on his right side since his stroke ten years ago. Today, I put him in his wheelchair to take him for a ride to the garden to see all the beautiful flowers when I noticed your father was staring intently at me! So I said, 'Al, are you trying to tell me something?' Your father got the biggest twinkle in his eyes and suddenly, he lifted his paralyzed arm up into the air and wiggled his fingers at me!"

She said the doctors were baffled; they had never seen any condition of paralysis show signs of improvement after ten years. I was as shocked as the nurse was. God's lavish love, by way of His plant oils, had far exceeded all of our expectations.

Shortly after that call, I was on an airplane to Iowa to witness this amazing recovery for myself. Before Dad's nurse would let me into his room, she asked me to describe how he looked the last time I saw him.

"His face was pasty white and his skin lacked any kind of vibrancy," I told her.

"Exactly," she replied. "Now go look at him!"

When I walked through the door, I thought I was in the wrong room! Dad's face was glowing, his cheeks were all pink, and his arms were almost pink with color.

I turned to the nurse. I asked, "What happened? What is this?"

"Oxygen!" she declared. "These oils are doing something to raise his oxygen levels."

They say seeing is believing and if the lavender oil that helped during my pregnancy wasn't enough to convince me of the benefits of essential oils, Dad's progress was.

With God, All Things Are Possible

Friend, when all seems hopeless and the future seems grim, think again! Nothing is impossible with God—nothing! Do not let the enemy of your soul convince you that your health is hopeless; you do have options. Your history does not have to be your destiny. Your body is designed to heal itself when given the proper nourishment, along with a positive attitude and prayer.

My father continued to show many signs of improvement, including more arm movements and a lot of grunting in an attempt to talk again. Dad could even sit in a wheelchair and beat me at checkers.

The one component we must always consider in any healing is the person's emotional state. The car accident had traumatized Dad, who was a very tender-hearted man, full of love for his family. He and Mom had a solid, loving marriage and he was also very close to Kathy, who intended to take over his business. Dad may have never fully recovered emotionally from losing them. So at age eighty-three, Dad went home to be with the Lord, his wife, and daughter. My brother, sisters, and I are so grateful that his last days were spent free of pain, colds, and flus. Dad left a legacy of tenderness and love that lives with us still.

Anointing for You and Your Family Today

What about you and your close circle of loved ones? How would it change your life if you could live in your best health ever? What would you love to do that you currently can't because of some physical limitation?

Prayer and anointing with oil are God's original design for your best health. Exercise, a good attitude, and healthy food choices are all part of the *therapeuo* or therapeutic healing process.

The wisdom in God's Word combined with the science behind essential oils makes a great tool for you and your family.

Perhaps you did not come from a family interested in good health. It's time to let go of some old ideas. Today is a new day and you have a chance to create a brand-new legacy, a new pattern for your next generation—one of longevity, vitality, and joy.

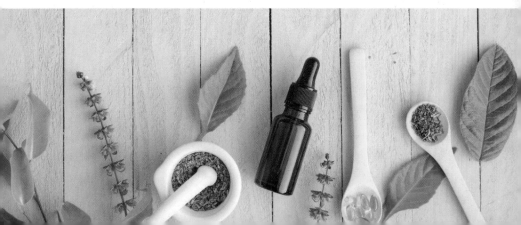

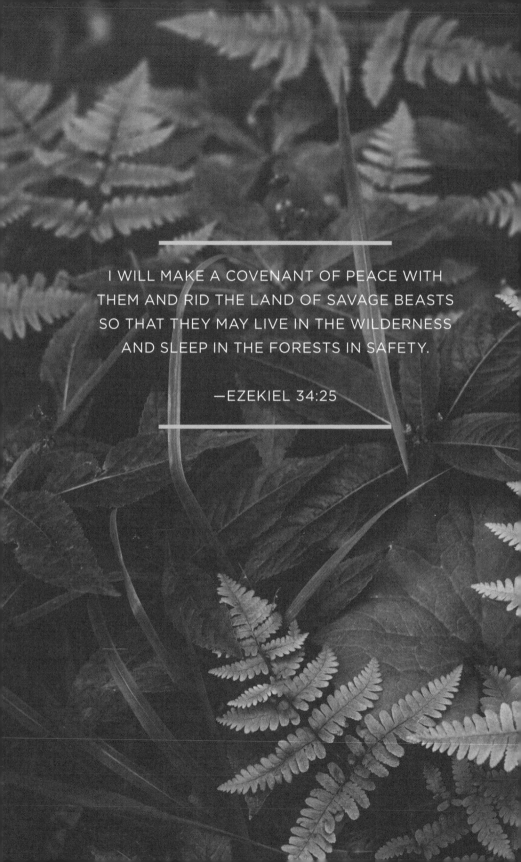

I WILL MAKE A COVENANT OF PEACE WITH
THEM AND RID THE LAND OF SAVAGE BEASTS
SO THAT THEY MAY LIVE IN THE WILDERNESS
AND SLEEP IN THE FORESTS IN SAFETY.

—EZEKIEL 34:25

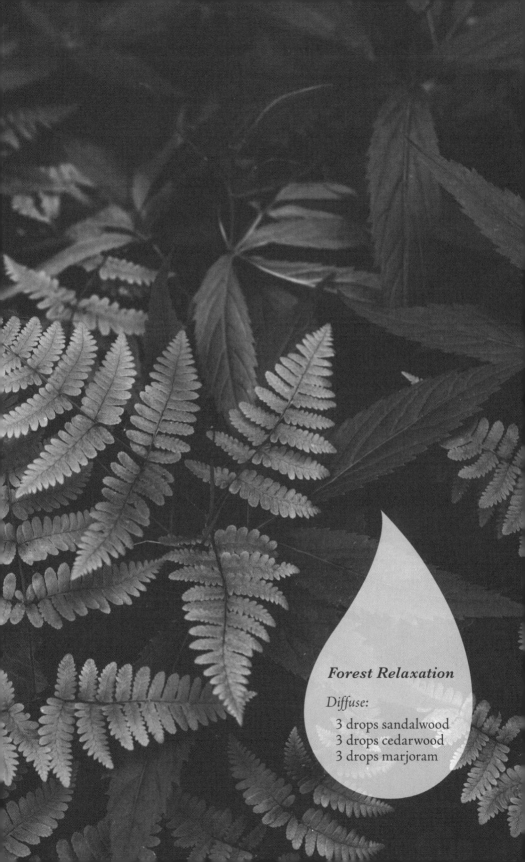

Forest Relaxation

Diffuse:

    3 drops sandalwood
    3 drops cedarwood
    3 drops marjoram

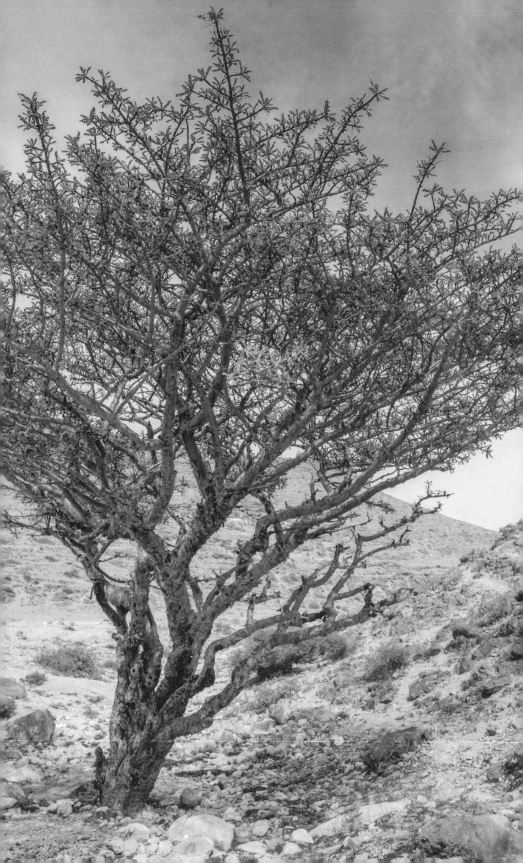

4

HOW DID QUEEN ESTHER CAPTURE THE HEART OF A KING?

W omen, how would you like to capture the heart of your "king"? Never underestimate the power of attraction when a woman is operating in her full gifts and potential. Queen Esther's alluring beauty and grace not only captured the heart of one man, but ultimately, her favor saved an entire nation.

Friend, if you have ever avoided reading the Bible because you thought it was boring, hold on to your hat! You are about to learn of the complex story of a beautiful Jewish orphan girl, a queen who gets banished, an illicit affair, a royal wedding, a lavish banquet, the highest form of betrayal, bravery at the risk of death, and a true love that lasts—all in one book of the Bible. Welcome to the story of Esther.

A quick overview of the story: Vashti, the wife of King Xerxes, dishonored her husband in front of many people. While Xerxes, also known as Ahasuerus, was hosting a grand seven-day feast, he wanted his guests to see his beautiful wife. Now, Vashti, who was also hosting a party of her own, refused to honor her husband's request. Thus the king, in his embarrassment and anger, decided to banish Vashti and choose a new wife. Yes, this was the culture of the times. The king made the rules.

A notice was sent across the land that all young, beautiful women were to be taken to the palace to be prepared to meet King Xerxes. But much was to take place before this meeting of destiny.

Among the maidens taken was a young Jewish girl known as Hadassah, which means Myrtle. Her cousin, who was her guardian, told her to go by the name of Esther to hide her identity.

Esther was entrusted to Hegai, the king's eunuch who was in charge of the harem. Because she pleased him and won his favor, she was immediately moved to the best part of the harem and given seven attendants from the king's staff. Those attendants were assigned to take care of her and oversee her beauty treatments and her food plan for the next twelve months.

Bathed in Precious Oils

Those first six months were devoted to beautifying Esther with the precious oil of myrrh. Imagine bathing in water scented with sweet-smelling myrrh oil and being anointed and massaged with myrrh oil every day for six months!

But it didn't end there. For another six months, Esther was prescribed special perfumes and cosmetic treatments. In other words, she was "marinated" in essential oils every day. Finally, after many months of preparation and purification, Esther's day of destiny arrived and she was presented to King Xerxes.

> *When the turn came for Esther... to go to the king, she asked for nothing, other than what Hegai, the king's eunuch who was in charge of the harem, suggested. And Esther won favor of everyone who saw her.*
> (Esther 2:15)

Before continuing the story, I want to emphasize something very important about essential oils: they do much more than just beautify the skin. They will affect every part of our being, including our body, our soul (mind, will, and emotions), and our spirit.

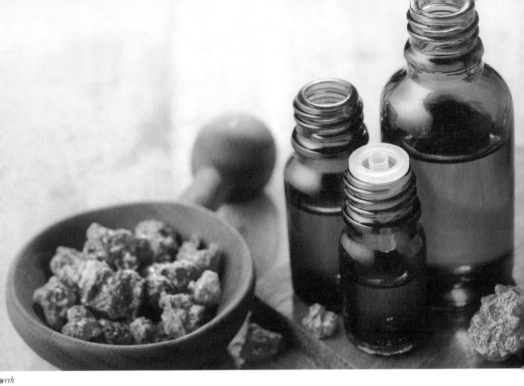

myrrh

Called to Save Her People

Esther was about to embark on the greatest calling on her life—the saving of her people from an evil plot to destroy the entire Jewish nation. For God to entrust this assignment to her, Esther had to be cleansed spiritually. She needed to be strengthened physically, as she was about to have intimate relations with a king who was very worldly and had been with many women before. Finally, she needed to be girded up emotionally; she needed maturity and strength to step into the position as the new Persian queen. While she already possessed great humility, she needed the confidence it would take to boldly approach the king at the risk of death to tell him about the plot to kill her people.

During the twelve months of Esther's preparation, those precious essential oils were absorbed through her skin and circulated into every cell of her body. As she inhaled their rich fragrances, they also reached the amygdala region of her brain, the seat of her emotions. She was radiantly beautiful on the outside. On the inside, Esther had been deeply cleansed, strengthened, and truly prepared for her calling. Take a look at the results:

Now the king was attracted to Esther more than to any of the other women, and she won his favor and approval more than any of the other virgins. So he set a royal crown on her head and made her queen instead of Vashti. And the king gave a great banquet, Esther's banquet, for all his nobles and officials. He proclaimed a holiday throughout the provinces and distributed gifts with royal liberality. (Esther 2:17–18)

The king was so joyful, so elated with Esther, that he generously gave out gifts to celebrate. Now that's a story!

Recently, I read John C. Maxwell's commentary on Esther's story, which emphasizes her significance in history:

"Esther joined the company of illustrious deliverers such as Joseph, who kept his people alive during the famine in Egypt; Moses, who led Israel out of slavery; Samson and David, who delivered the Hebrews from the Philistines; and Gideon, who delivered the people from the hand of

Frankince

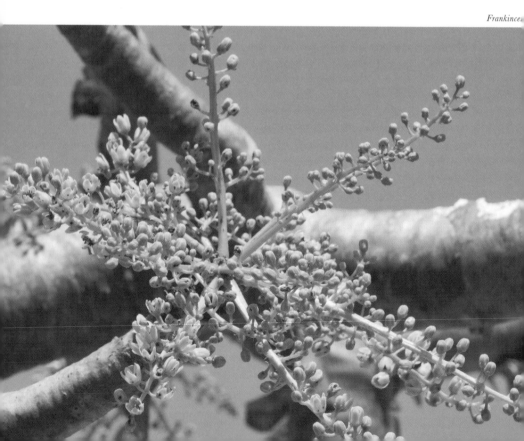

the Midianites. Esther tells the story of an ordinary person who fulfills an extraordinary leadership challenge in an unlikely context. She is a Jew in a foreign land and a woman in a male-dominated world—a minority within a minority. But God raised her up at exactly the right time."[25]

Never underestimate the influence of a woman who walks in humility yet keeps herself bathed in the fragrance of the Lord. And never underestimate a woman who is well-loved.

What is it about myrrh oil that causes it to be the most-mentioned precious oil in Scripture? The stories of myrrh oil are full of romance, mystery, and intimacy.

One Bible commentary notes, "Fragrant perfumes were an indispensable mark of royal gratification to the kings of Persia, which were burnt before them whenever they went abroad; and it is most likely, therefore, that fondness for cosmetics led to the purification ritual described in Esther. In fact, perfumes were used profusely, without regard either to cost or to quantity."[26]

Myrrh and frankincense perfumed King Solomon's own magnificent procession as he made his way to his bride. Sitting in a gold and silver coach, Solomon was surrounded by sixty of his finest soldiers. Thick pillars of smoke arose from swinging incense burners as they traveled, a sacred sacrifice to God and a royal honor to Solomon's new queen, the Shulamite, who is thrilled at the sight.

> *Who is this coming out of the wilderness like pillars of smoke, perfumed with* **myrrh** *and* **frankincense**, *with all the merchant's fragrant powders? Behold, it is Solomon's couch, with sixty valiant men around it.... Go forth, O daughters of Zion, and see King Solomon with the crown with which his mother crowned him on the day of his wedding, the day of the gladness of his heart.*
>
> (Song of Solomon 3:6–7, 11 NKJV)

For sheer romance, leaving a love note of sweet-smelling myrrh on the door latch has to be at the top of the list.

I rose up to open to my beloved; and my hands dropped with myrrh, and my fingers with sweet smelling myrrh, upon the handles of the lock. (Song of Solomon 5:5 KJV)

It was a custom among some ancient peoples to anoint doors used by a bride with fragrant oils, which helps us to understand this verse more readily. In his Enduring Word commentary, Davis Guzik wrote: "As the maiden finally rose from bed and came to the door, she noticed that the door or the latch of the door had been anointed with sweet perfume. This was another reminder of the beauty and the quality of his love for her."[27]

There are seventeen references to myrrh in the Bible, with eight in the Song of Songs. Here are two from other books:

All your robes are fragrant with myrrh and aloes and cassia; from palaces adorned with ivory the music of the strings makes you glad. (Psalm 45:8)

I have perfumed my bed with myrrh, aloes and cinnamon. (Proverbs 7:17)

Myrrh Use in History

Myrrh was widely used by the Arabian people for soothing sunburned, dry, cracked skin. It is said that Greek soldiers would not go into battle without a poultice of myrrh for their wounds.

Since ancient times, frankincense and myrrh have been burned in places of worship to uplift spirits and enhance contemplation. However, it serves a hygienic purpose as well, purifying the air and reducing any less-than-desirable smells. In one test, burning incense reduced airborne fungus and bacteria by more than 80 percent.[28]

Myrrh is such a thick oil, it's almost like honey. This is why it's such an exquisite skin oil. It is also uplifting, refreshing, and restoring. When my chest feels tight, I love to apply myrrh and enjoy quick, soothing relief. Living near the ocean and walking barefoot on the beach daily, I often have dry heels, which I easily correct with myrrh essential oil.

When I think of all the money I spent in past years on skin care, make-up, and hair care, the price of pure, therapeutic myrrh, with all of its health and beauty benefits, seems very reasonable. I think both frankincense and myrrh will become two of your favorite oils for your family's natural medicine cabinet.

Treatment for Soft, Thick Hair

Since moving to Doha, Qatar, near the Persian Gulf, I have become *very* interested in the oils of ancient Scripture. After a couple of months in the hot, dry weather here, I noticed a change in my skin and hair. My hair was falling out and had become dry and brittle. It was shocking. So right away, I mixed drops of myrrh, spikenard, cedarwood, and sandalwood in a cup of olive oil and covered my hair and scalp with it. After two hours, I shampooed my hair. Wow, I couldn't believe the difference! My hair was soft again!

I use this treatment once a week on my hair now. It has stopped falling out completely and has become thicker and softer. All of my friends here are asking me for my oil treatment now. As for my skin, myrrh and spikenard are a great addition to my ART skin care for the extra moisture. I am so grateful for quality essential oils!

—*Carolyn Watts, Doha, Qatar*

Hair Treatment Recipe:

1/2 cup of olive oil
5 drops *each* of
myrrh, sandalwood, cedarwood, and spikenard essential oils

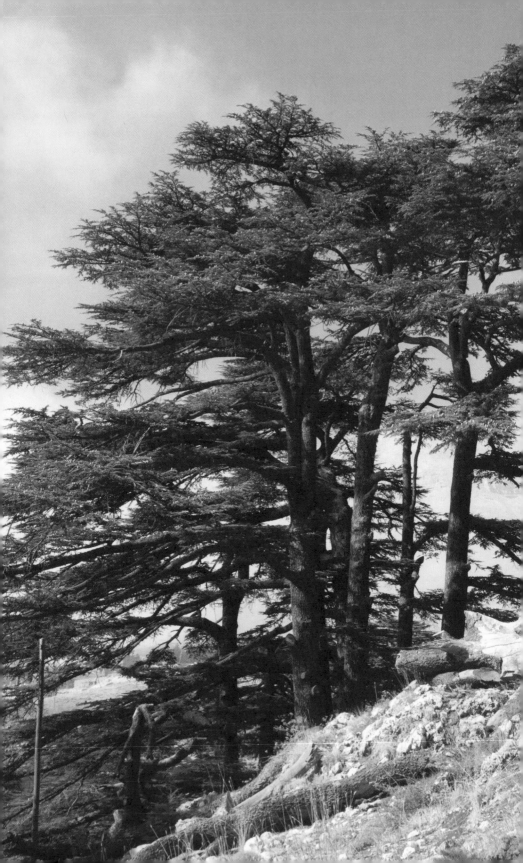

5

WHAT DID KING SOLOMON
KNOW THAT WE NEED
TO KNOW?

The "bigger than life" story of King Solomon reveals two amazing essential oils from the *Who's Who* of the essential oil world and the tremendous impact they had on everyday life during his reign.

Solomon became the king of Israel around the age of twenty in 971 B.C. after his father, David. While David was a man of war, Solomon was a man of peace. At the beginning of his reign as king, Solomon made one request of God:

> *Now, LORD my God, you have made your servant king in place of my father David. But I am only a little child and do not know how to carry out my duties. Your servant is here among the people you have chosen, a great people, too numerous to count or number. So give your servant a discerning heart to govern your people and to distinguish between right and wrong. For who is able to govern this great people of yours?*
>
> (1 Kings 3:7–9)

God was delighted by Solomon's request because he hadn't asked for long life, wealth, or the death of his enemies. So the Lord granted Solomon great wisdom. In addition, God lavishly poured out on him honor, wealth, and a promise of long life *"if you walk in obedience to me and keep my decrees and commands"* (1 Kings 3:14).

My fascination with this story began about three years ago as I was writing my first book on this subject, *A Biblical Perspective on Essential Oils*. Because the Lord had been wooing me to write on this topic for a long time, my desk had a considerable stack of research and notes on it. But the Lord spoke to my heart and said I was missing an important part of the story. I reviewed all of my information, but could not ascertain what I had overlooked. Finally, I just said, "Please tell me, Papa, what am I missing?"

He lovingly replied, "You are missing the story of My son, Solomon."

As I dove into the story of Solomon, my heart just leapt! On the pages before me, I discovered the queen of Sheba and the immeasurable, lavish gifts she brought to Solomon, including expensive spices. I learned of a glorious architectural structure never before seen on the face of the earth, designed and built by Solomon. I discovered a king totally sold on God's plan and purpose for his life. And then I found a man who, toward the end of his days, forgot who he was and was led wildly astray by his 700 wives.

But the most riveting thing I learned was that Solomon was a botanist. He had deep knowledge and understanding of the earth, trees, and plants. So what did Solomon know that we need to know? What did he learn that we need to learn?

The Wisdom of King Solomon

God gave Solomon wisdom and very great insight, and a breadth of understanding as measureless as the sand on the seashore. Solomon's wisdom was greater than the wisdom of all the people of the East, and greater than all the wisdom of Egypt. He was wiser than anyone else.... And his fame spread to all the surrounding nations. He spoke three thousand proverbs and his songs numbered a thousand and five. He spoke about plant life, from the cedar of Lebanon to the hyssop that grows out of walls. He also spoke about animals and birds, reptiles and fish. From all nations people came to listen to Solomon's wisdom, sent by all the kings of the world, who had heard of his wisdom.

(1 Kings 4:29–34)

First, we see that Solomon spoke 3,000 proverbs, some of which we still have today in the book of Proverbs. Next, we discover that he wrote 1,005 songs. What a surprise to learn this great king was a composer, too.

The first book of Kings also tells us that Solomon talked about trees and plants—apparently everything from the mighty, towering cedar tree to the small, flowering hyssop plant. We also learn that he gave lectures on animals, birds, reptiles, and fish, but these are mentioned after Solomon's knowledge of botany. There are hints elsewhere of some of Solomon's wisdom, such as when he mentions apples (see Proverbs 25:11) and pomegranate (see Song of Songs 4:3). In fact, there are references to nature throughout the beautiful, sensual Song of Songs.

Since people *"from all nations"* came *"to listen to Solomon's wisdom,"* there has to be something important there for us to discover. Let's start with the cedar tree.

dar

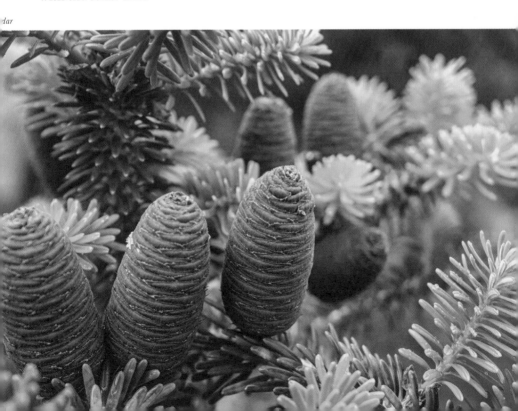

Cedar

The mighty cedars of Lebanon were known for their towering strength and longevity; these magnificent trees are said to live up to 2,000 years. Cedar wood was highly desirable for building in ancient Israel due to its extreme durability, fine grain, attractive yellow color, fragrance, and resistance to insect damage. Even today, chests made out of cedar are prized for storing blankets, pillows, and other textiles.

King David used cedar wood in building his palace. His son used cedar to build the first temple in Jerusalem and his own palace.

It's thrilling to read about all of the intricacies of the building of Solomon's temple and the different places cedar wood was incorporated into the design. (See 1 Kings 6:1–38, 7:13–51; 2 Chronicles 3:1–15, 4:1–22.) The temple walls were lined with cedar planks featuring carved figures of cherubim, palm trees, flowers, and gourds.

It's no surprise that there is much more to this tree than just wood for building. Cedar wood essential oil is even more valuable in everyday life now.

Ce

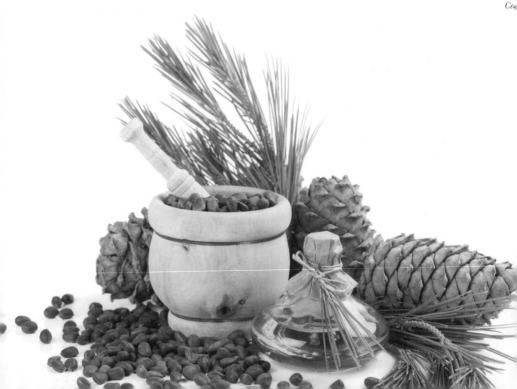

Cedarwood Essential Oil

Cedarwood essential oil is derived from the bark of the cedar tree and is believed to be the very first oil ever distilled. Today, it's a widely-used, multipurpose essential oil that's inexpensive compared to rare oils like frankincense and spikenard. It is mentioned twenty-five times in eight different books in the Bible.

Here are eight reasons to keep cedarwood oil in your home:

1. Better Brain Power

This oil contains a natural chemical compound that gives it the ability to cross over the blood-brain barrier and oxygenate the limbic region of the brain, which controls essential human behavior. Cedarwood oil offers unlimited potential in the area of mental acuity, memory function, and support.

A study conducted by the late Dr. Terry S. Friedmann found that children with attention deficit and hyperactivity disorder (ADHD) could greatly improve their focus and learning capacity by breathing in cedarwood oil. Thirty-four children with ADHD were given one of three essential oils (cedarwood, vetiver, or lavender) to smell three times a day for thirty days. At the end of the study, the researchers found that thirty children in both the vetiver and cedarwood oil groups experienced improvements in brain activity and reduced the ADHD symptoms.[29]

2. A Good Night's Sleep

Another valuable component of cedarwood oil is natural melatonin. Breathing in a few drops thirty minutes before bed or diffusing it at your bedside can be very relaxing and promote a good night's sleep.

Here's a great example from my own life. One afternoon, while preparing for a radio talk show appearance, I began breathing cedarwood oil, as I am so attracted to its woodsy smell. Before I knew it, one of my children was waking me up because I had fallen sound asleep sitting at my desk. Ever since then, cedarwood has become one of my "must have" travel oils for long airplane flights and unfamiliar hotel rooms. With just a couple of drops on the bottoms of my feet and a few drops on my pillow, I am literally out like a light.

3. A Great Fragrance for Men

Attention, men: cedarwood oil, with its soothing, woodsy scent, is a very popular component of men's cologne. If you're a do-it-yourself kind of guy, try adding a drop or two to a little olive oil and apply behind your ears and on your wrists or underarms. Now you can enjoy a pure cologne with no chemicals, additives, or fillers—just pure, intoxicating oil! As a woman, I love smelling cedarwood oil on a man. It's very masculine and supporting.

4. No More Hair Loss

Consider trying my favorite recipe for healthy hair and scalp: mix together two drops cedarwood essential oil, two drops rosemary essential oil, and two drops lavender essential oil. Add two ounces of olive oil and mix gently. Apply to your scalp and massage it in. Leave it in for a minimum of thirty minutes or put on a shower cap and leave in overnight, then shampoo it out. Use every other day for thirty days. An added benefit is the rosemary essential oil supports your memory function.

5. Banish Anxiety

How did Solomon keep up with the needs and personalities of his 700 wives? Perhaps he had massive diffusers filled with cedarwood essential oil running 24 hours a day. Cedarwood offers beautiful support for your emotions and helps to keep you calm. If you're feeling anxious, try this: several times a day, place a few drops of cedarwood oil in the palms in your hands, cup them around your nose, and breathe in deeply.

6. Clears Up Congestion

When you start to feel congested, pour a few drops of olive oil into your hand, add a few drops of cedarwood oil, and rub this on your chest.

7. Keep the Insects Away

Cedarwood is your must-have oil during the summer months. Wherever and whenever you notice insects, it's time for cedarwood. Diffuse into your home and office. Add to a spray bottle with water and spritz as needed. Cedar chips are often placed in closets or chests because they repel moths and other insects. For fleas and ticks, dilute cedarwood oil with olive oil and massage into your pet's fur if your veterinarian gives their approval. You can also keep pests off of you and your family with this mixture.

8. Acne Away

The purifying properties of cedarwood oil make it helpful for pimples, blackheads, and whiteheads. Dilute with a few drops of olive oil before applying on a problem area. Leave on for ten to fifteen minutes, then remove with your cleanser.

What Did Solomon Teach About Hyssop?

Hyssop is a brightly colored shrub in the mint family with white, pink, or blue blooms. In ancient times, hyssop leaves were used to make a strong tea to help those with nose, throat, and lung infections.

This powerful essential oil, along with cedarwood, was required in an Old Testament cleansing ritual for those with leprosy. (See

ssop

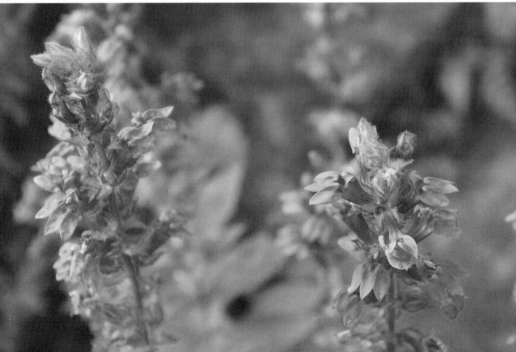

Leviticus 14:4–6.) Some Bible scholars relate this use to a verse in one of the Psalms: *"Cleanse me with hyssop, and I will be clean; wash me, and I will be whiter than snow"* (Psalm 51:7).

The most widely known story about hyssop oil involves a dramatic rescue operation for the people of Israel. The hard-hearted pharaoh, ruler of Egypt, refused to let the Israelites leave the land, so God was about to bring judgment down upon his house for his continued cruelty. The Israelites had been held captive in Egypt for 430 years. Here are the instructions that the children of Israel received:

> *Take a bunch of hyssop, dip it into the blood in the basin and put some of the blood on the top and on both sides of the doorframe. None of you shall go out of the door of your house until morning. When the LORD goes through the land to strike down the Egyptians, he will see the blood on the top and sides of the doorframe and will pass over that doorway, and he will not permit the destroyer to enter your houses and strike you down.* (Exodus 12:22–23)

There are two pivotal points here. First, when the angel of death saw the blood on the top and sides of the door, he was not allowed to enter the house. Second, when you take a hyssop branch and strike the post, oil is released. This powerful and cleansing oil comforted the people and protected them from harm. The angel of death literally "passed over" every Israelite home thus marked. This was the origin of the Jewish festival of Passover.

The Benefits of Hyssop Oil

1. Promotes a Healthy Respiratory System

As an expectorant, hyssop can help to loosen phlegm that can become deposited in your respiratory tract. The antispasmodic nature of hyssop helps to relieve spasms in the respiratory system and it's soothing for a cough. Singers, teachers, and others who use their voice a lot may greatly benefit by diluting hyssop with olive oil and massaging it on the throat area.

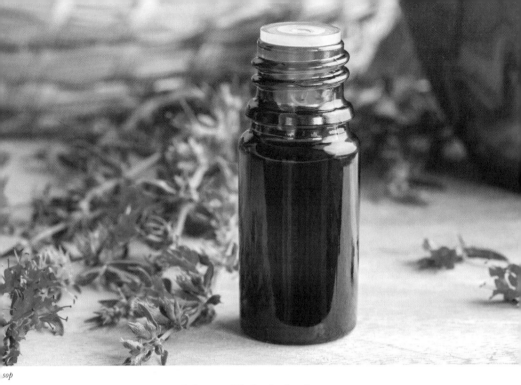
sop

2. Helps to Fight Infections

The antiseptic properties of hyssop make it a good choice to apply to a wound or cut. Some studies show that hyssop may be effective in lowering plaque formation for patients with genital herpes, a chronic infection that is sexually transmitted.[30] (When using hyssop oil topically in this way, always dilute with olive oil or coconut oil.)

3. Increases Circulation

Simply put, our bodies need to have good circulation to be healthy. When our blood flows freely throughout our body the way God intended, you can see a decrease in swelling and inflammatory response. To soothe swollen ankles, apply a few drops of hyssop to the ankles and massage the legs upward toward the heart. Hyssop's ability to improve circulation may also help to alleviate hemorrhoids.

4. Supports Healthy Digestion

Hyssop helps to stimulate the production of secretions of stomach acid, digestive enzymes, and bile. As food makes its way to the stomach, these gastric juices break down food for digestion. Hyssop also helps the body to absorb nutrients and encourages the removal of gases from the intestines, thus reducing indigestion, nausea, loss of appetite, and heartburn.[31]

To promote proper digestion, mix a few drops of hyssop essential oil with olive or coconut oil and massage onto the lower abdomen. As an alternative, diffuse hyssop oil throughout a room or keep a bottle handy to sniff throughout the day.

5. Promotes Healthy Skin

Hyssop helps to promote cellular regeneration and the growth of new skin. As an antiseptic, it helps to kill bacteria and may be beneficial in fighting acne. It can also be used to diminish the look of scars from stretch marks or wounds.

Biblical Oils for a New Generation

Just imagine: these same oils and many more that were used in biblical times have been rediscovered for this generation to keep us strong in body, soul, and spirit. God's love is everlasting and his provision for us is lavish.

Now you have two more vital essential oils to add to your family's natural medicine chest, cedarwood and hyssop.

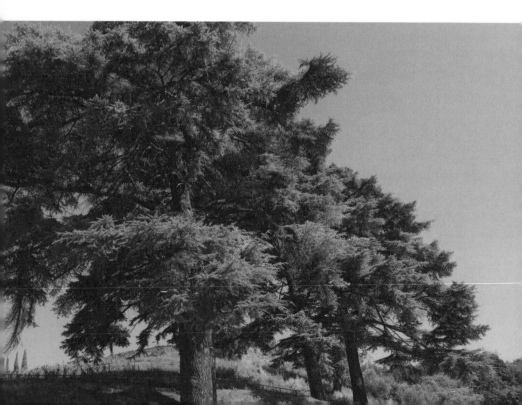

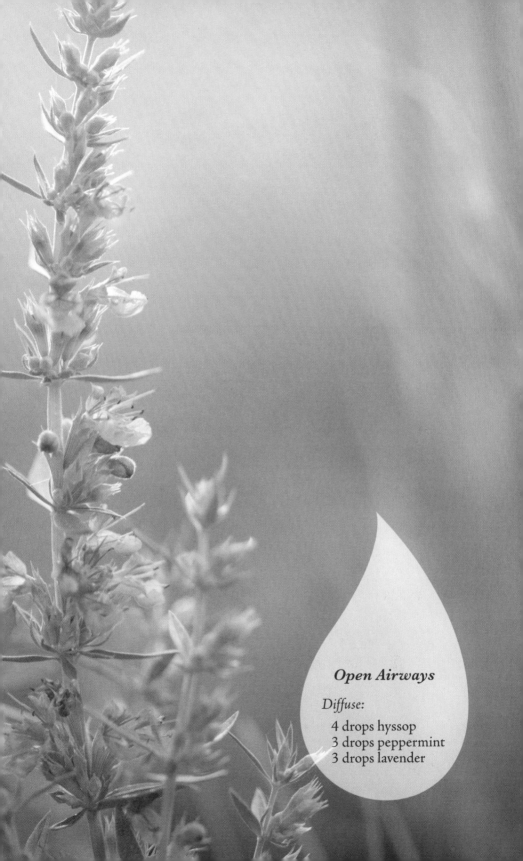

Open Airways

Diffuse:

  4 drops hyssop
  3 drops peppermint
  3 drops lavender

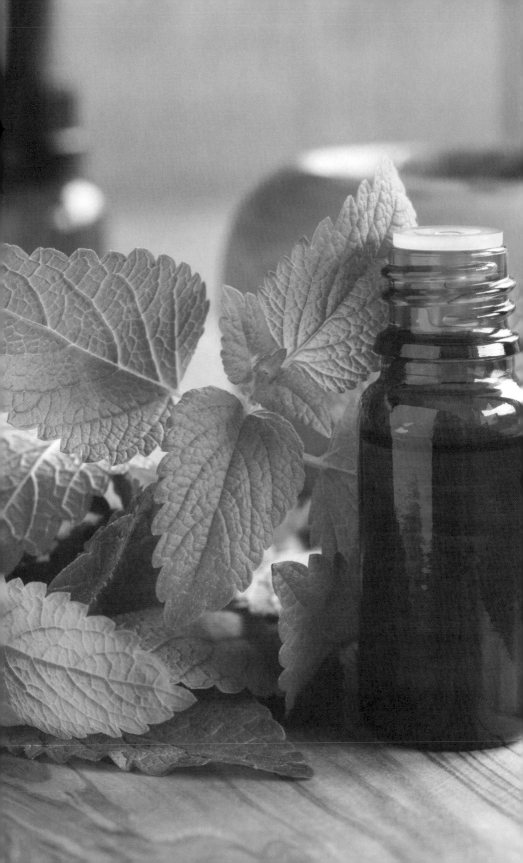

6

SUPPORTING EACH SYSTEM OF YOUR BODY

The intricate blueprint of your body is nothing short of miraculous. When God designed us, He gave us twelve unique systems designed to strongly carry us into each stage of our lives. While each system is unique, they are interdependent on each other. When one system is out of balance, the others are affected. This is why you should avoid treating the symptoms of an illness and instead be intentional about supporting your body as a whole.

The chemical structure of essential oils is so complex that many of them work on more than one body system. Two essential oils in particular—frankincense and lavender—are considered to be "universal" in that they support nearly every system in the body. When in doubt about which oil to use, these are your go-to oils.

If we examine the systems of our body and the benefits of various essential oils, we can see that God gave us plants to support each system.

I must stress that this information should not be used to diagnose or treat any medical condition; it's meant for educational purposes only. Be sure to work with your doctor or medical professional as you add essential oils to your health routine.

How to Choose Essential Oils

As a certified wellness coach, I have had the privilege of living in Europe for five years and traveling the world for the past twenty-five years while investigating essential oils. While there is no industry standard for grading oils, I use the term "supplement-grade" to distinguish essential oils that are pure enough to be taken internally.

The labels on these oils will include a notification that the oil may be taken as a supplement and will suggest a serving size. Never exceed the amount suggested on the label unless directed to do so by a healthcare professional. Always work with your doctor or medical professional and seek their advice before starting an internal routine of essential oil.

How to Select a Brand

When selecting an essential oil brand, look for a company that is a reputable, reliable source of essential oils. A company that controls the entire life cycle of the plant—planting, harvesting, distillation, and bottling—will take the utmost care to preserve the delicate, health-supporting capabilities of the essential oil.

To produce premium essential oils, the source plants, flowers, and trees should be grown in healthy soil without pesticides and herbicides; harvested precisely at their peak; either cold-pressed or steam-distilled at low temperatures to preserve their therapeutic value; and carefully sealed in dark bottles.

What about Essential Oil Blends?

Many companies produce essential oil blends to support specific needs in the body. Blends combine several single oils in a way that can be beneficial.

In this chapter, you will learn about many powerful single oils. As your essential oil knowledge increases, I encourage you to branch out and learn more about essential oil blends.

12 Body Systems and Essential Oils

The human body's twelve distinct systems perform specific functions that are reflected in their names: cardiovascular, digestive, endocrine, immune, integumentary, lymphatic, muscular, nervous, reproductive, respiratory, skeletal, and urinary. Some essential oils are particularly useful for certain systems.

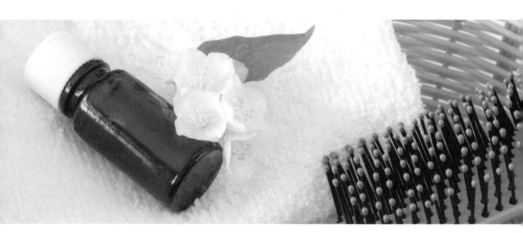

Integumentary System

This system includes your hair, skin, and nails. It also includes your sweat glands, which allow your body to regulate your body temperature.

+ **Frankincense** is great for easing acne, reducing large pores, and tightening the skin. It also reduces the look of fine lines and wrinkles. Add three drops to your daily face cream.

+ **Rose** hydrates dry skin, clears up acne, reduces signs of aging, minimizes the appearance of scars, and helps with conditions such as eczema and rosacea.[32] It's naturally moisturizing, too. You can apply two to four drops of rose oil directly to the area you need it or dilute with a pure almond or coconut oil.

+ **Myrrh** has been found to heal skin conditions such as athlete's foot and eczema and aid in wound healing.

+ **Lavender** evens out skin color and tone. It also calms and sooths skin irritated by the sun, heat, or insect bites. (However, if you are allergic to insect venom and are bitten by a hornet, spider, and the like, you should seek medical help immediately.) Lavender can be applied directly to skin that's been irritated by an insect bite. You can also add two drops to your daily face moisturizer. For sunburn or overheating, mix ten drops of lavender in one ounce of distilled water and use a glass misting bottle.

+ **Cedarwood** has been known to reduce and treat hair loss by increasing blood flow to the scalp; it may also promote hair growth.[33] Combine five drops with a carrier oil such as olive or with chemical-free shampoo and massage it into the scalp. Let it sit on the scalp for ten minutes and then rinse out.

+ **Cypress** helps to prevent acne caused by toxins in the diet or skin care products. Place three drops of supplement-grade cypress oil into an empty capsule and fill with olive oil or almond milk. Take with food up to three times daily. Cypress has also been known to reduce the appearance of cellulite. Massage two or three drops of cypress over the area of concern in circular motion for one minute twice a day.

+ **Myrtle** provides astringent properties for oily skin and can tighten sagging skin. Add three to five drops to a daily face cream or body cream. Increase to up to ten drops if no change is seen after seven days.

+ **Spikenard** cleans and brightens the skin. Apply two to four drops to your daily facial cleanser. To support hair growth, add fifteen drops of spikenard to your shampoo; rinse after five minutes. Be careful not to let any get into your eyes because it may sting.

+ **Sandalwood** is a natural skin exfoliator, so it's helpful when fighting acne while reducing fine lines and wrinkles. Add two to four drops to your daily moisturizer.

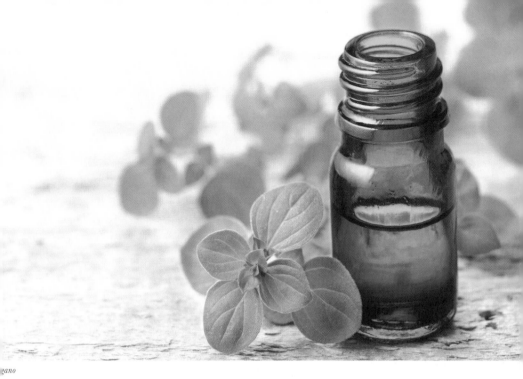

gano

Immune System

Protecting your body from illness, the immune system consists of the lymph nodes, spleen, thymus, and bone marrow.

+ **Frankincense** increases the blood's white cell count, which helps to fight infection. Place three drops of supplement-grade frankincense oil into an empty capsule and fill with olive oil or almond milk. Take with food up to three times daily.

+ **Oregano** kills unhealthy bacteria, which is key in boosting your immune system. A little goes a long way with this oil. Too much can cause stomach issues and cause the skin of the affected area to feel hot. Place one or two drops of supplement-grade oregano into an empty capsule and fill with olive oil or almond milk. Take with food up to twice a day. Oregano can also be massaged on the bottoms of the feet. Dilute two to four drops into a tablespoon of virgin unrefined coconut oil and rub over the chest and neck. Be sure to spot test a small area for sensitivity.

+ **Hyssop** supports the immune system's ability to fight infections. It also promotes warming for patients with a cough and shivering fever.[34] Combine one part hyssop essential oil with one part virgin unrefined coconut oil and rub over the chest as well as the front and back of the neck.

+ **Helichrysum** has "free-radical scavenger properties."[35] This means it helps to protect your cells from the damage caused by free radicals, which are unstable molecules that can build up in your cells and increase the risk of cancer and other diseases. To take advantage of the benefits of helichrysum, it's best to take this essential oil internally. Place four drops of supplement-grade helichrysum oil into an empty capsule and fill with olive oil or almond milk. Take with food once a day.

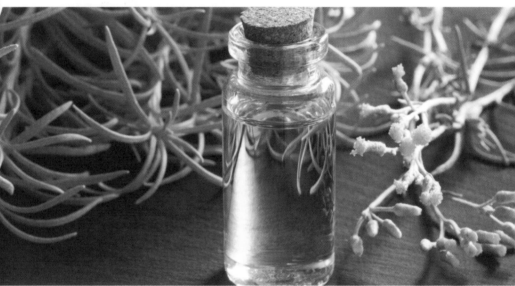

Helichry

Cardiovascular or Circulatory System

This system includes your heart, blood, arteries, veins, and capillaries. It's responsible for the flow of nutrients and oxygen throughout your body as well as hormones to and from cells. It is also moves waste away from the cells.

+ **Helichrysum** naturally reduces blood pressure. Massage three drops of helichrysum oil over your heart and rub one or two drops on your left hand, one inch below your ring finger.

- **Ginger** warms the skin, which promotes good circulation—a key factor in healing wounds. Mix two to four drops into virgin unrefined coconut oil and massage. Repeat as necessary.

- **Cypress** has been known to remove toxins from the body while contracting veins and promoting healthy blood flow. Place three drops of supplement-grade cypress oil into an empty capsule and fill with olive oil or almond milk. Take with food up to three times daily for detoxification. For veins, place two to four drops over the needed area and massage. Dilute if needed. To promote healthy circulation, place two to three drops on feet and ankles and massage upward toward the heart.

- **Ylang-ylang** has been known to regulate heartbeat. Apply two to four drops over the heart area and massage. Dilute if needed.

- **Frankincense** is effective against atherosclerosis, a chronic inflammatory disease which causes heart disease.[36] To use topically, place one to three drops of frankincense on the soles of each foot and massage in; place a drop one inch below the ring finger on the left hand and massage in. To take internally, place three to four drops of supplement-grade frankincense into an empty capsule and fill with olive oil or almond milk. Take with food up to once a day.

- **Lavender**'s soothing properties have been known to help with hypertension. Apply two to four drops over the heart area, or diffuse up to three times daily.

- **Basil** supports healthy arteries and limits the buildup of bad, low-density lipoprotein (LDL) cholesterol. Rather than using dried basil when cooking, try supplement-grade basil essential oil. Less than a drop can usually flavor a whole pot of tomato sauce or soup. See chapter 7, Creative Cooking With Essential Oils.

- **Juniper** aids in healthy blood circulation. Apply two to four drops directly to the affected area.

- **Bergamot** may lower cholesterol levels[37] and has been shown to decrease blood pressure and heart rate.[38] Place three to four drops of supplement-grade bergamot into an empty capsule and fill with olive oil or almond milk. Take with food up to three times daily.

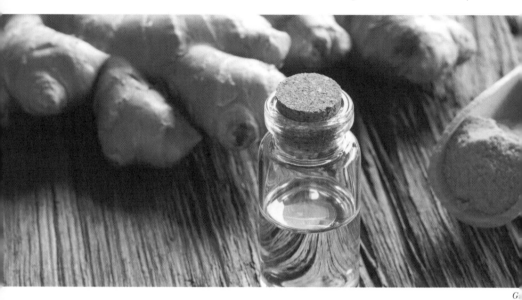

G

Digestive System

Designed to digest foods, liquids, and other consumed substances and absorb their nutrients, this system consists of the tongue, esophagus, oral cavity, pancreas, large and small intestines, anus, liver, and salivary glands.

+ **Peppermint** supports healthy daily digestion. Use topically by rubbing one or two drops over the stomach area or mix one drop of supplement-grade peppermint in a glass of water. Drink before a meal for extra support. Peppermint essential oil has also been shown to soothe irritable bowel syndrome.[39] Place three drops of supplement-grade peppermint essential oil into an empty capsule and fill the rest with coconut oil. Take one capsule twice a day for at least four weeks.

+ **Hyssop** supports a healthy liver and gallbladder while also soothing general intestinal discomfort. It has also been known to disperse gas, increase appetite, and soothe colic. Apply two to four drops over the stomach area, intestines, or abdomen as needed.

+ **Myrtle** can be soothing to hemorrhoids. Add five to six drops to one ounce of scent-free, dye-free cream and apply after every bowel movement as needed.

+ **Ginger** has been shown to be effective in soothing nausea, particularly during pregnancy.[40] Apply two to four drops over the stomach area for relief. Place two drops into the palms of your hands and breathe deeply until the symptoms abate. You may also diffuse up to sixty minutes for ongoing relief.

+ **Tarragon** has been known to be a diuretic and alleviate excess water retention in the body. Dilute 50/50 with your favorite carrier oil and apply two drops over the abdomen area.

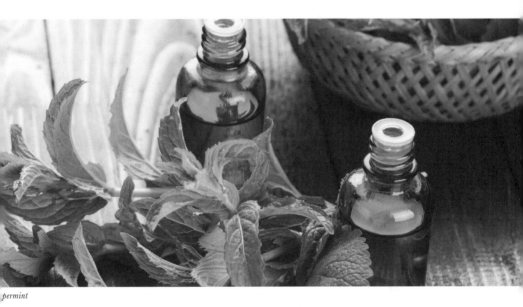

permint

Endocrine System

This system is responsible for all of our hormones. It consists of the pituitary, pineal, thyroid, and adrenal glands, the pancreas, and the endocrine part of ovaries (in females) and testicles (in males). It also includes the parathyroid glands—four tiny glands in the neck, each about the size of a grain of rice, that allow the body to properly absorb calcium.

+ **Spearmint** supports the health of the parathyroid glands. Rub one to two drops over the neck as needed.

+ **Geranium** promotes healthy estrogen and progesterone levels in women. Place two drops over the ovary area twice daily.

+ **Lavender** supports the pineal gland, which is responsible for healthy sleep patterns. Diffuse five to ten drops of lavender at night in a cold air diffuser to receive its calming benefits for a restful sleep. You can also consider taking a soaking bath twenty minutes before bedtime. Place five to ten drops into the bottom of a bathtub and fill with warm water.

+ **Lemongrass** supports a healthy, balanced thyroid gland. Massage one drop over the front and sides of the neck for daily support.

+ **Frankincense** supports the pituitary gland, which is often considered the "master gland" as it helps all other endocrine glands function well. Place two drops of frankincense into the palms of your hands and breathe deeply for one to five minutes at least once a day to support your endocrine system.

+ **Rosemary** supports the pancreas, which controls healthy blood sugar levels, and the adrenal glands, which are responsible for our stress responses. Rosemary essential oil on the skin can provoke a hot response so dilute it 50/50 with virgin unrefined coconut oil and apply it over the pancreas area for maximum support. To alleviate stress, use supplement-grade rosemary essential oil to replace dried herbs in recipes you already make. (See chapter 7, Creative Cooking With Essential Oils.)

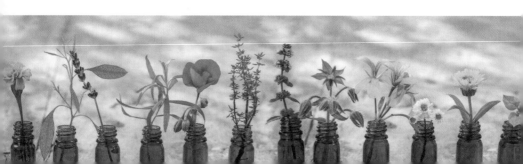

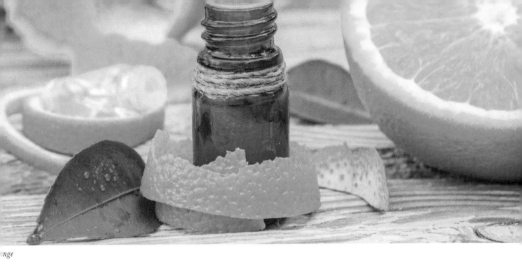

Skeletal System

The skeletal system includes your bones, of course, but also your joints and teeth. The latter are the hardest part of your body even though they are not bones. The skeletal system works closely with your muscular system to help you move. Your bones provide structure, cartilage, and ligaments to allow your muscles and organs to connect. This system also protects your organs.

- **Peppermint** is ideal for broken bones. Has been shown to reduce discomfort from injuries as well as flush out fluids that can build up around a bone injury. Dilute 50/50 and apply as close to the affected area as possible as needed.

- **Clove** has been used for centuries to soothe tooth discomfort. Apply topically where needed. Test a small area first as clove can be a very warm oil. Dilute as needed.

- **Orange** and **Ginger** have both been shown to reduce joint discomfort and stiffness while also increasing physical function.[41] Massage two to four drops of the preferred oil over the needed area twice daily. Dilute as needed.

- **Frankincense** reduces the periodontal inflammation that causes gingivitis.[42] Add two drops of frankincense essential oil to your toothpaste when brushing.

- **Wintergreen** stimulates bone repair while calming irritated tissue due to injury. Apply two to four drops over the needed area. Never place oil into an open cut.

- **Pine** has been shown to prevent bone loss.[43] Place three drops of supplement-grade pine oil into an empty capsule and fill with almond or coconut oil, or almond milk. Take up to three times per day.

- **Helichrysum** reduces discomfort and aids in bone repair. Apply two drops at the base of the neck and down the spine, and massage one drop on the bottom of each foot three times a day. Also apply over the affected area or as close as possible to the area three times a day.

- **Lemongrass** has been found to be effective in soothing joint swelling and stiffness. Apply two to four drops of oil to the area and massage up to five times each day.

- **Chamomile** has been known to soothe discomfort in inflamed joints. Apply two to four drops of oil to the area and massage up to five times a day.

Cyp

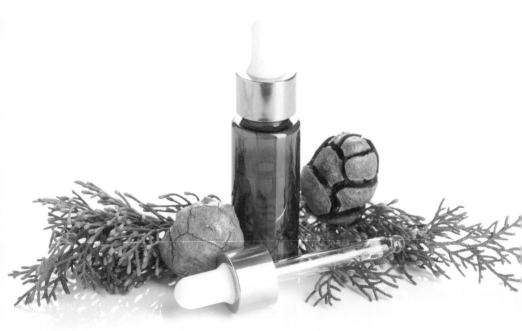

Lymphatic System

An important part of your immune system, the lymphatic system filters out bacteria and manages body fluid levels. It consists of your lymph nodes, lymph vessels, spleen, tonsils, adenoids, and thymus.

+ **Frankincense** supports the overall health of the lymphatic system. Place three drops of supplement-grade frankincense into an empty capsule and fill the rest it with olive oil or almond milk once daily. Apply two drops over lymph nodes as needed.

+ **Myrrh** cleanses the lymphatic system. Apply two drops over lymph nodes as needed.

+ **Cypress** helps the body remove excess water and salt that can lead to fluid retention. Massage two to four drops over ankles and on your left palm about an inch below your thumb.

+ **Peppermint** increases the movement of lymph fluid and helps the lymph nodes flush. It is also very soothing to swollen nymph nodes. Apply two drops over lymph nodes as needed.

+ **Oregano** has been known to dissolve buildup in the lymph system. It's most effective when taken internally. Place two drops of supplement-grade oregano into an empty capsule and fill the rest of the capsule with olive oil or almond milk. Take up to three times per day.

Muscular System

The muscular system works with your skeletal system to help your body move. It consists of smooth and cardiac muscles, skeletal muscles, and tendons.

+ **Peppermint** is soothing to muscles, particularly after working out or some other strenuous activity. Dilute 50/50 with the carrier oil of your choice and apply on the affected area as needed.

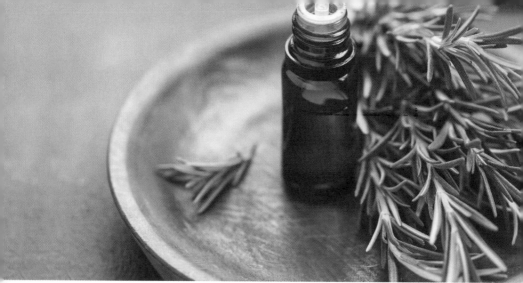

- **Juniper** eases tension and soothes muscle spasms. It may be used undiluted by applying one to three drops on location; reapply as needed.

- **Lemongrass** works to strengthen weak muscles, ligaments, and connective tissue. It also soothes sore muscles. Dilute one drop of lemongrass oil with four drops carrier oil and apply over the affected area before, during or after workout. Apply as needed.

- **Marjoram** relaxes tight muscles and muscle tension. It has also been known to help soothe tendonitis. Apply two to four drops to the needed area.

- **Rosemary** is helpful for easing discomfort and inflammation. Apply two to four drops to the sore or inflamed area.

- **Wintergreen** soothes muscle tension after exercise. Apply two to four drops where it's needed.

- **Frankincense** has been known to soothe muscles and tendons. It can be used undiluted by applying one to three drops on location; reapply as needed.

- **Helichrysum** is effective in soothing chronic muscle or tendon discomfort. It can be used undiluted. Apply one to three drops on location three to five times a day.

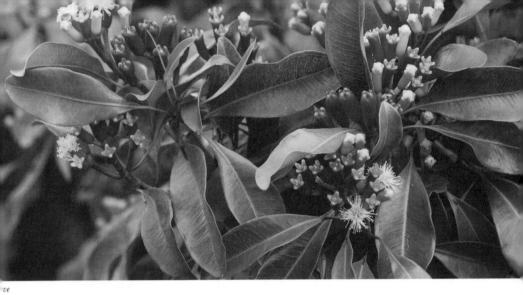

+ **Chamomile** has been known to soothe discomfort in tendons. Apply two to four drops of oil to the area and massage up to five times each day.

Nervous System

Coordinating body functions, the nervous system consists of the brain, spinal cord, nerves, and nerve endings.

+ **Juniper** boosts nerve regeneration. Apply two to four drops topically over the needed area.

+ **Lemongrass** stimulates nerves, thus helping to send signals throughout the body and to the brain. Apply two to four drops topically over any area in need, such as the spine or any place where you feel a pinched nerve.

+ **Frankincense** protects nerve endings are supports nerve regeneration. Apply two to four drops topically over the needed area.

+ **Clove** has a chemical compound that has been shown to be effective at restoring nerve function in those with diabetic neuropathy.[44] Dilute clove 50/50 with the carrier oil of your choice and apply over the affected area three times daily.

+ **Helichrysum** has been known to regenerate nerves in the ear and testing has begun to dewtermine its effect on spinal cord nerves. *Warning: never place essential oils inside your ears!* Instead, you may apply two drops behind the ear and around the ear twice daily. You may also place a few drops on a cotton ball and place it outside the ear while you sleep.

+ **Geranium** has been known to soothe aching nerves while it speeds healing. Apply two to four drops to the area as needed.

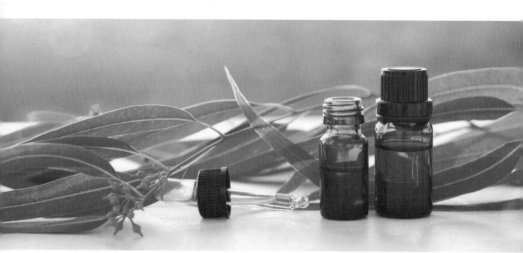

Eucalyptus Radia

Respiratory System

This system consists of your nose, trachea, lungs, bronchioles, bronchi, alveoli, and alveolar sacs. It breathes in air, absorbs oxygen into the bloodstream, and breathes out carbon dioxide.

+ **Cedarwood** is soothing to the bronchial tubes. Place five to ten drops in a cold air diffuser and diffuse up to an hour. For more immediate relief, place two drops into the palms of your hands, cup them over your nose and mouth, and breathe deeply for two to five minutes.

+ **Cistus** is an expectorant and can dissolve thick mucus. Place five to ten drops in a cold air diffuser and diffuse up to sixty minutes. Or place four to five drops into a bowl of steaming water, cover your head with a towel, and breathe in the soothing vapors.

+ **Eucalyptus Radiata** has been known to dilate the trachea in both people and pets. Place five to ten drops in a cold air diffuser and diffuse nightly. You can also apply two to four drops over the chest and neck for soothing relief.

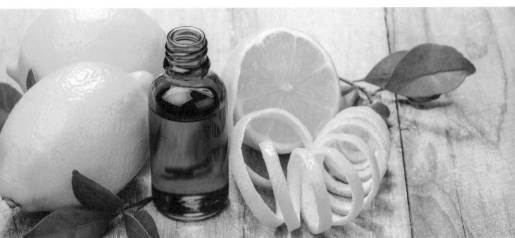

non

+ **Frankincense** strengthens and supports lung function.[45] Take a palliative bath by placing five to ten drops into the bottom of the tub and filling with warm water. You may also diffuse five drops for thirty to sixty minutes or place two to three drops over the chest and lungs to soothe the respiratory system.

+ **Hyssop** has been known to be an expectorant, loosening excess phlegm trapped in the lungs and respiratory tract. Place five to ten drops in a cold air diffuser and diffuse up to an hour.

+ **Myrtle** has been known to open the lungs and sinuses. Place five to ten drops in a cold air diffuser and diffuse up to an hour, place one or two drops on a clean finger and swipe under the nose. You may also dilute 50/50 and apply to the neck and chest as needed.

+ **Ravensara** is soothing to the entire respiratory tract. Place five to ten drops in a cold air diffuser and diffuse up to an hour.

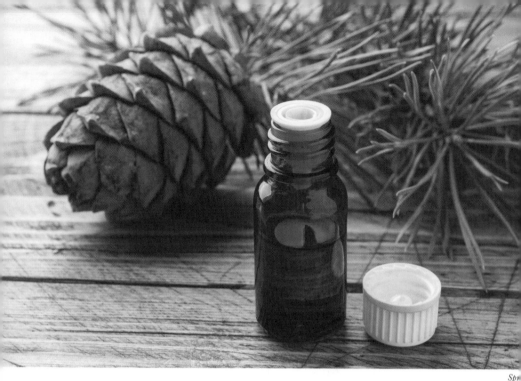

- **Wintergreen** is milder than myrtle and has been known to open the lungs and sinuses. Place five to ten drops in a cold air diffuser and diffuse up to an hour, or place one or two drops on a clean finger and swipe under the nose. You may also dilute 50/50 and apply to the neck and chest as needed.

- **Cypress** is soothing to the respiratory system. Place two to four drops over the chest and neck for soothing relief.

- **Spruce** has been known to dilate bronchial tubes. Place five to ten drops in a cold air diffuser and diffuse as needed. You can also apply two to four drops over the chest and neck for respite.

- **Lemon** should be used at the first sign of the sniffles. It has been known to strengthen white blood cells that can support your body's health. Dilute 50/50 in a carrier oil and rub over chest and neck up to five times a day. *Warning: lemon is photosensitive so cover up these areas if you will be out in the sun.*

Urinary System

The main function of the urinary system is removing urea (a type of waste) from your blood. Consisting of your bladder, kidneys, and urethra,

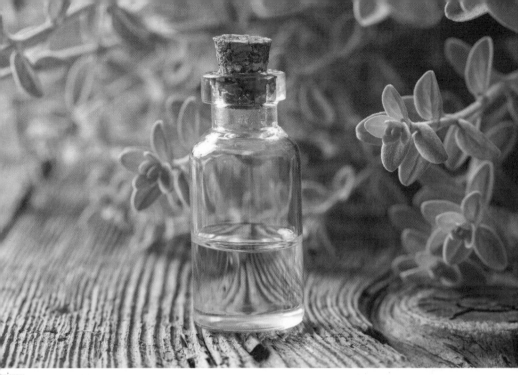

this system can be prone to bacteria. For good health, it's important that this system functions correctly.

+ **Clove** is known to kill bacteria that can live in the bladder. Place three drops of supplement-grade clove oil into an empty capsule and fill with olive oil or almond milk. Take with food up to three times a day.

+ **Oregano** supports healthy bacteria levels in the urinary tract. Place three drops of supplement-grade oregano oil into an empty capsule and fill with olive oil or almond milk. Take with food once daily.

+ **Cinnamon** has been known to balance bacteria in the urinary system that could prevent infections there from recurring. Place three drops of supplement-grade cinnamon oil into an empty capsule and fill with olive oil or almond milk. Take with food up to once a day for maintenance.

+ According to a 2013 study, the following essential oils support a healthy urinary system: sage, basil, rosemary, marjoram, and hyssop. Select the oil of your choice from this list, dilute 50/50 in carrier oil, and rub over the bladder area.[46]

Reproductive System

The reproductive system consists of the vulva, ovaries, uterus, clitoris, and labia for females, and the penis and testes for males. Addressing the benefits of essential oils for this system, our goal is hormonal balance and fertility. Some of these oils can be used by both men and women.

Female Reproductive System: Hormone Balancing

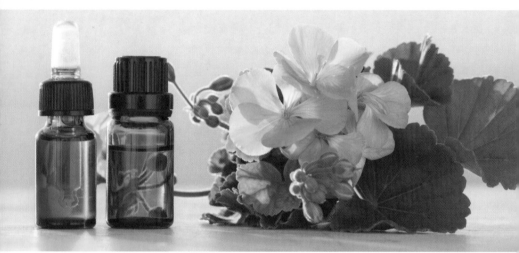

Geranium

- + **Frankincense** has been known to reduce stress and enhance thyroid function, which can support healthy hormone balance. Place one drop of supplement-grade frankincense under your tongue each morning.

- + **Geranium** naturally balances hormones and its pleasant scent is very relaxing. Place two drops on the inside of each ankle every night and morning to balance hormones. Diffuse five to ten drops for twenty to sixty minutes each day to take advantage of its stress-relieving properties.

- + **Clary Sage** has been known to reduce cortisol levels and improve thyroid hormone levels to help with stress that can throw off healthy hormones. Place two drops on the inside of each ankle every night and morning.

+ **Bergamot** has been known to soothe hormonal imbalance caused by emotional stress. Place two drops of supplement-grade bergamot oil in a mug and add hot water and your favorite herbal tea. Diffuse five to ten drops for twenty to sixty minutes daily.

+ **Myrtle** helps regulate menstrual cycles. Apply two to four drops over the lower abdomen just before and during cycles, three to five times a day.

+ **Peppermint** has been known to cool hot flashes. Apply one drop to the back of your neck. Avoid if you have high blood pressure.

Female Reproductive System: Fertility

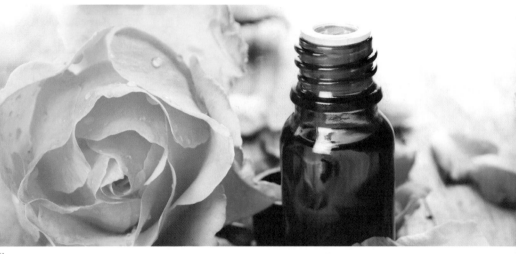

+ **Geranium** promotes healthy estrogen and progesterone levels as well as healthy eggs. Place two drops over the ovary area twice a day.

+ **Clary Sage** has been known to increase female libido. Apply one drop to the inside of each ankle every night.

+ **Rose** promotes libido in women and has been known to improve cervical mucus. Place two to four drops over the ovary area twice daily.

+ **Ylang-ylang** energizes the reproductive organs and balances hormones. It has been known as an aphrodisiac for centuries. Diffuse five to ten drops in a cold air diffuser twenty to sixty minutes before passion. Place two to four drops on the lower abdomen daily. Use as a perfume on the wrists and neck.

Male Reproductive System: Hormone Balancing

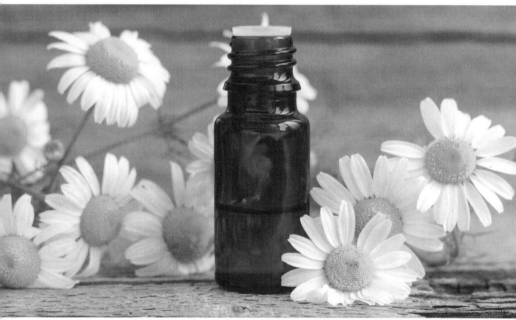

Chamor

+ **Rosemary** removes excess estrogen from the body. Apply one drop to the outside of each ankle every night.

+ **Frankincense** has been known to reduce stress and balance thyroid function to promote healthy hormone balance. Place one drop of supplement-grade frankincense essential oil under your tongue daily.

- **Bergamot** has been known to soothe hormonal imbalance caused by emotional stress. Diffuse five to ten drops in a cold air diffuser twenty to sixty minutes daily.

- **Chamomile** lowers cortisol hormone levels. Place two drops in the palms of your hands and cup over your nose and mouth. Breathe deeply for five minutes.

Male Reproductive System: Fertility

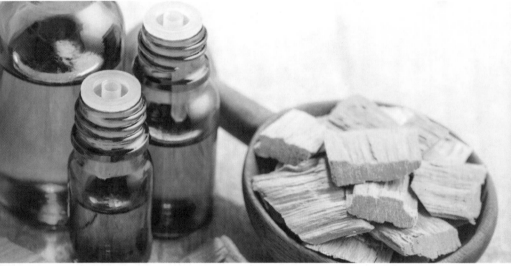

ndalwood

- **Sandalwood** ignites the sexual desires of a man and has been known to raise testosterone levels. Place five to ten drops into a diffuser and begin diffusing twenty minutes before passion is to be awakened. Use as a cologne on the wrists and neck daily.

- **Rose** helps improve sexual dysfunction and performance anxiety. It has also been known to increase sperm count. Apply two to three drops over the lower abdomen and rub in daily.

- **Frankincense** has been shown to increase sperm count.[47] Apply two or three drops over the lower abdomen and rub in daily.

+ **Goldenrod** boosts male libido and had been known to help with impotence. Place two to four drops on the lower abdomen and inner thighs. *Caution: do not place oils on sensitive areas.*

+ **Ylang-ylang** energizes the reproductive organs and balances hormones; it has been known as an aphrodisiac for centuries. Diffuse five to ten drops in a cold air diffuser twenty to sixty minutes before passion. Place two to four drops on the lower abdomen daily.

Golden

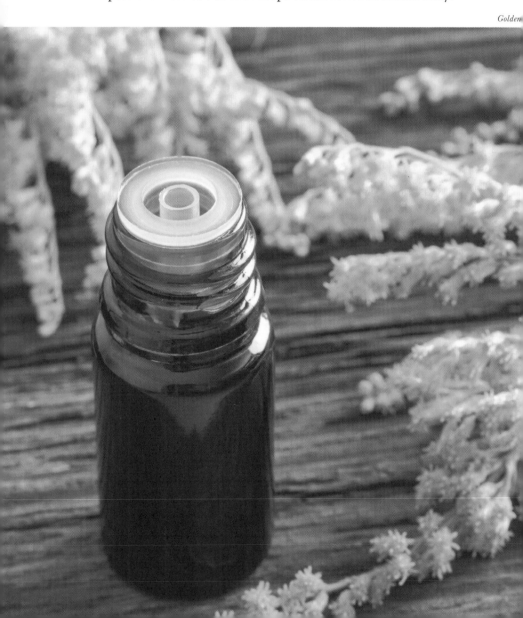

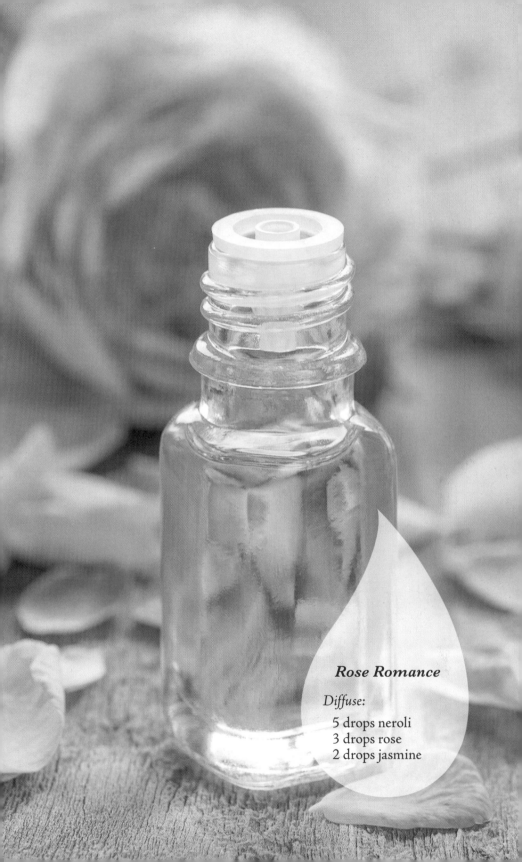

Rose Romance

Diffuse:

5 drops neroli
3 drops rose
2 drops jasmine

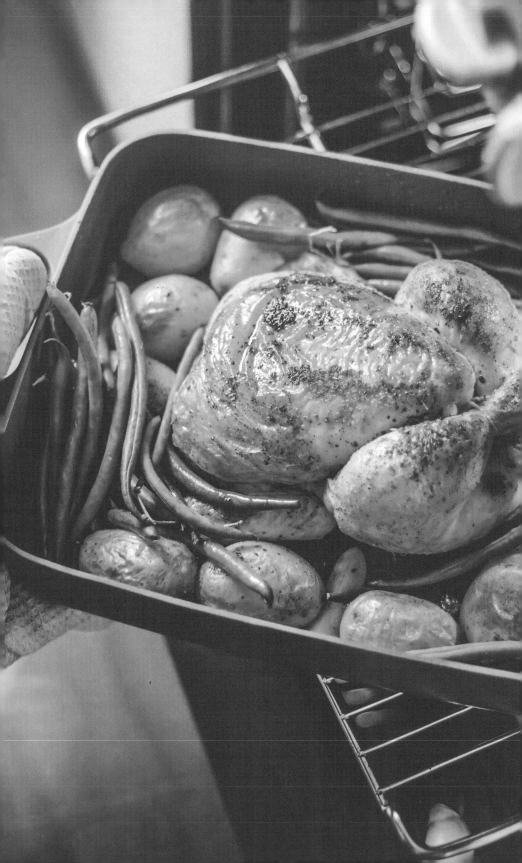

7

CREATIVE COOKING WITH ESSENTIAL OILS

W hether you're a picky eater, foodaholic, or a food connoisseur, you have to eat to live.

We had a saying in our family: "Every good memory starts and finishes with food." Since most of us eat two or three times a day, why not enjoy something delicious? Eating can be a celebration!

Dad, my four siblings, and I really appreciated Mom's creative gift with food. She could take the most boring tuna casserole and make it taste like a five-star, gourmet extravaganza. And most of the time, when Mom cooked, she sang, which brought us even more joy.

At age fifty-five, our mom turned her love of cooking into a highly successful French cooking school. Our dad was so proud of Mom that he would come home from his business just to peel dozens of potatoes to help her prep for a class.

Well, if you're like me, you reach a point somewhere in your life where you wake up one morning and think, "Ugh! I am so sick of all my recipes that I cannot cook another meal."

That's exactly how I felt for about the first thirty-five years of life. You see, even though Mom had a thriving cooking school, I wanted nothing to do with the kitchen.

Growing up, I was a tomboy and the outdoors was always calling me. My sweet dad taught me how to ride horses and my love of riding brought me infinitely greater pleasure than being "stuck in the kitchen."

There was only one problem: once I got married and had children of my own, I realized we were all going to starve to death if I did not change my attitude. So, if you are bored to tears with your recipes—or maybe you don't even like to cook—but realize the health of your family is at stake, take heart. There is hope.

Essential oils to the rescue!

Cooking with essential oils adds punch, zest, and complex flavors to your food. And the best part is you are creating a new legacy of forward-thinking, delicious nutrition for your family.

Never in a million years did I think my children would call me "hip," yet that is what I hear them tell their friends about me now. Having fun in the kitchen as a family is one of the most life-giving memories you will create

Joseph making p

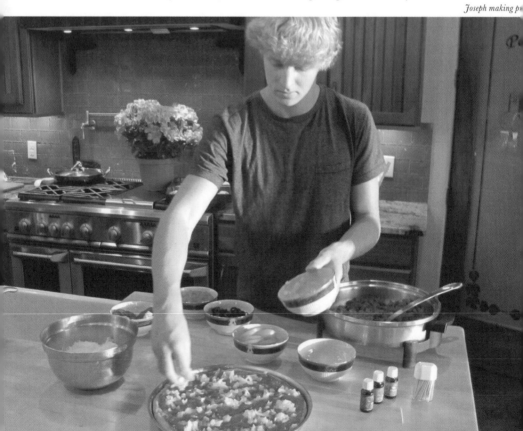

with your loved ones. Essential oils can give your "humdrum" recipes an instant lift and entice many people into your kitchen with the scents and tastes.

My Personal Health Journey

Allow me to share my own journey back to optimal health so you can see why it is critical to fall in love with good foods as a way of life.

While growing up, almost everything we ate was either organic or natural. We had an organic garden and if you did not help out with weeding, pruning, watering, and harvesting, you did not eat. Period. However, our parents had a way of making it fun. We were encouraged to try vegetables and fruits as we were harvesting them at their peak ripeness—everything from sweet green peas to big, succulent strawberries. Mom made an angel food cake topped with just-picked strawberries that was heavenly! And on hot summer days after working in the garden, my sisters and I would throw on our swimsuits, race down to the lake, and jump right in off of the dock.

iel cooking

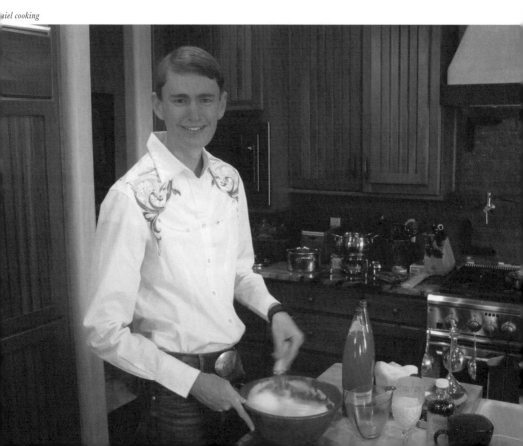

Several nights a week, Mom and Dad would make gigantic bowls of homemade popcorn—no microwave stuff for us!—and hand-squeezed orange and grapefruit juice. The five of us kids would sit around the dining room table, doing our homework, snacking on popcorn, and drinking fresh juice. The time our parents put into hand-squeezing that juice still amazes me. They set an example of love and joy that continues to inspire us today.

Another favorite foodie memory I have is making doughnuts from scratch. Every Sunday morning, Mom would invite people over for brunch after church. Anyone who did not have somewhere to go came to our home. Dad and I were the official doughnut-hole makers of the family. Outside on the patio, come rain or shine, our operation was in full swing. We rolled them, dipped them, and covered them in every kind of unhealthy frosting imaginable. Of course, everyone loved them.

What I Didn't Know Did Hurt Me

There is one thing about health that none of us were aware of in those days: we had no idea about the health hazards of delicious, highly processed, highly addictive white sugar. Even though my family was eating wonderfully healthy meals, we also ate sugar in and on just about everything you can imagine.

As a result, by the time I was twenty years old, I was completely addicted to white sugar and chocolate. I developed hypoglycemia—a blood sugar imbalance—which took many years to diagnose and overcome. If I ate a candy bar just before getting in the car to drive somewhere, I was in real danger of falling asleep before reaching my destination.

In my mid-twenties, I began to undergo a series of very expensive tests to see what was wrong with me, but the doctors never could figure it out. The amazing thing is that no medical professional ever asked me what I ate!

Finally, in desperation, I went to a health food store and stayed there an entire day, reading books to see if I could find the answer. I did, in a very simple book entitled *Sugar Blues* by William Dufty.[48] I read the book cover to cover; every symptom the author described fit my situation to a "T." If you have low energy, high stress, mood swings, and weight gain, you might just have the "sugar blues," too.

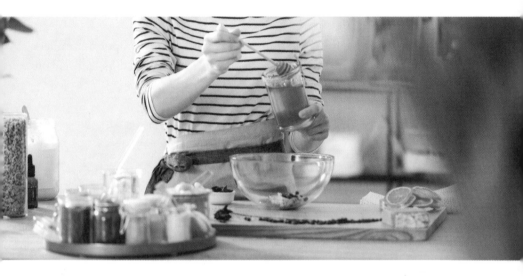

Hope for Your Sweet Tooth

Eliminating white processed sugar from my diet and replacing it with healthy sweeteners from God's garden turned my whole life around. Be encouraged! It wasn't that difficult. I found sweeteners that taste great and yet are not overprocessed or harmful. An added benefit was my slim figure reemerged after removing white sugar from my diet. Yours can, too.

If you feel that you're just getting by as far as your health is concerned, imagine feeling on top of the world instead. Your body is so miraculously made, that once you have the knowledge, avoid the things that are hurting you, and make better choices, your body actually heals itself rather quickly.

Most of us were not taught this in school, yet today, the knowledge is everywhere if you are looking for it. Good health isn't everything...but life is so much better with it. God put you on this earth to do a job and you might as well feel good while you're doing it.

Every day, we choose life or death with our forks. Shocking, isn't it? If I put a slice of succulent, ripe orange in my mouth, I am adding life to my body. If I eat a piece of calorie-laden, sugary pie instead, I am hastening my body's march toward death.

It really is this simple. Our choices are healing us or killing us, one bite at a time.

Sugar directly affects our emotions as it leaches out important minerals from our bodies. The answer is to change our eating habits, not rely on any drug.

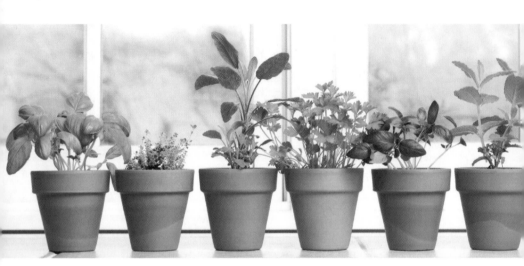

Live Foods vs. Dead Foods

Foods that still carry the essence and vitality of the plant they came from are "live" foods. They are foods in their most natural state, right off the tree or out of the garden. Live foods have vitamins and minerals that are critical to maintain a healthy body and mind.

On the other hand, "dead" foods are foods that have been overcooked or overprocessed, or have added preservatives, food coloring, artificial flavors, high-fructose corn syrup, mono and diglycerides, cellulose gum, and other ingredients that don't come directly from nature.

Consider live foods to be your friends. Here are some examples of foods that have life in them that can add life to you:

Live Foods

- Ripe, raw organic fruits and vegetables
- Lightly steamed or stir-fried vegetables
- Whole grains
- Dried beans and legumes
- Organic eggs, poultry, meat, and fish
- Raw or lightly roasted nuts and seeds
- Raw organic milk (not homogenized)
- Cultured milks such as kefir and plain yogurt
- Organic honey from your region
- Organic maple syrup and maple sugar
- Organic coconut milk and juice
- Pure organic oils, including coconut, grapeseed, olive, walnut, and avocado

Dead Foods

- Refined white sugar
- Most canned foods
- Overcooked foods
- White flour
- White pasta
- Foods with preservatives
- Foods with unpronounceable ingredients
- All butter substitutes
- Hydrogenated oils
- Foods with artificial food coloring

Does this mean we need to eat an all-raw diet? Of course not. Learn to listen to your body. Depending on your digestive system, some people do better with slightly steamed or cooked foods. But whichever way your body prefers food, it's time to kick the fast-food restaurant habit and get back into the kitchen.

Essential oils are not the cure-all in your kitchen. The cure-all starts in the grocery store or in your own garden, where you can choose fresh, healthy foods first. Then, essential oils will expand the flavors and the nutritional profile to extraordinary levels.

Drinking in God's Bounty

Step one to feeling great is to drink more water. Your body is made up of 55 to 60 percent water; your cells thrive on it.

One of the best ways to encourage your family to drink more water is to add the delicious flavor of essential oils to it. Some stellar essential oils you can enjoy in water are lemon, lime, grapefruit, orange, tangerine, and peppermint. Try one or two drops in a glass of water or five to six drops in an entire pitcher of water, or to taste. Just a single drop of peppermint oil is enough for an entire pitcher of water.

We like to put essential oils in our water pitcher and store it in the fridge to enjoy throughout the day. Try a different essential oil every day.

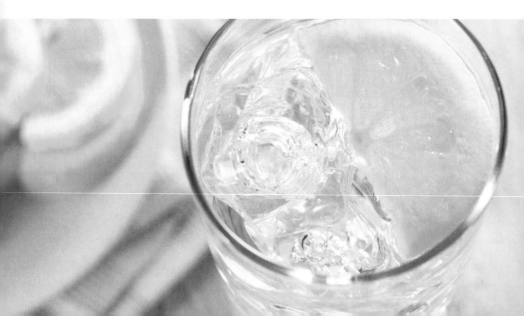

Citrus Essential Oils

Numerous studies show these oils contain high levels of *d-limonene*, a natural chemical constituent that offers several health benefits, including helping to support healthy cellular regeneration and relieving heartburn. Since orange essential oil has the highest concentration of d-limonene, consider drinking it in your water on a daily basis just for prevention purposes. Lemon essential oil makes a great, natural liver cleanser.

Peppermint Oil

Peppermint oil cools the body down in the summertime heat. It can also be your first defense against stomach and digestive weakness. For troubleshooting a tummy ache, add one or two drops of peppermint oil to a cup of warm water, stir well, and sip.

In addition, many doctors are now studying the effects of breathing peppermint oil to increase mental clarity and memory function.

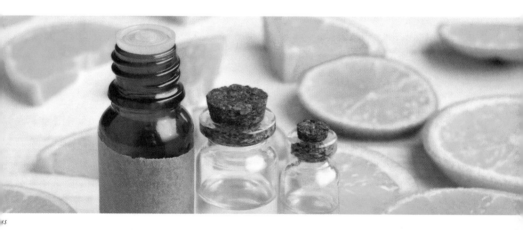

Creative Cooking with Essential Oils

For me, entertaining is euphoric. I'm so glad that having guests over for a meal doesn't have to mean preparing everything so that it's ready for them when they arrive. Half of the fun and pleasure is all being in the kitchen together—stirring, tasting, talking, and catching up. Then there are the table settings…oh là là! Dim the lights and create an alluring atmosphere with candles.

My children will tell you that I love any excuse to celebrate. Our gatherings often end up with dancing. Somehow, I just believe there has to be a ballroom in heaven where we will all be waltzing one day.

Consider cooking and eating a grand adventure—and it's your artistry that will make it happen.

When you add essential oils to your recipes, you are literally adding the life force of the plant itself. French physician Dr. Jean-Claude Lapraz taught me that it's important to create a terrain inside our bodies to make them an undesirable host for disease. We can do this through the life-giving foods we eat, especially foods enhanced with essential oils.

The most important principle to keep in mind when preparing foods with essential oils is "less is more." Essential oils are extremely economical to use in cooking because you use less than one drop of oil for most recipes. I literally start by dipping the end of a toothpick into the bottle and then stirring the toothpick into my pot of soup, stew, or casserole. I recommend that you let your dish cool a bit before you add the essential oil, so that the food retains more of the plant nutrients.

Savory essential oils complement main dishes and vegetables from Mediterranean, Thai, and Italian cuisines. Just think of every herb you currently use in your cooking and know, "There's an oil for that!" This includes basil, oregano, thyme, black pepper, lemongrass, rosemary, celery seed, marjoram, sage, dill, tarragon, and more.

I've included a few of my favorite recipes here so you can experience the flavor for yourself. For a complete book of recipes using essential oils, please see my book, *Eating Out of Heaven's Garden*.[49] You can also transform your own favorite recipes by replacing any dried herbs with essential oils.

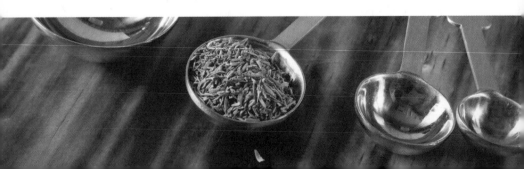

Approximate Herb to Oil Equivalents

1 tablespoon dried herbs is similar to one drop of essential oil

1 teaspoon dried herbs is similar to one toothpick of essential oil

Start with the toothpick and add more to taste. Remember the old cooking adage, "You can always add more, but you cannot take it away."

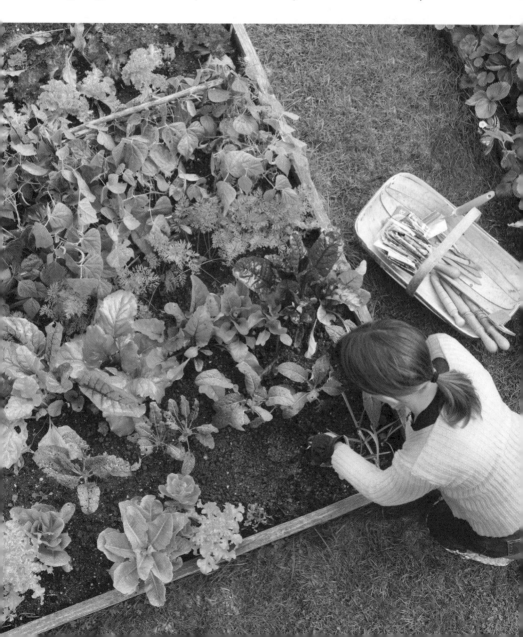

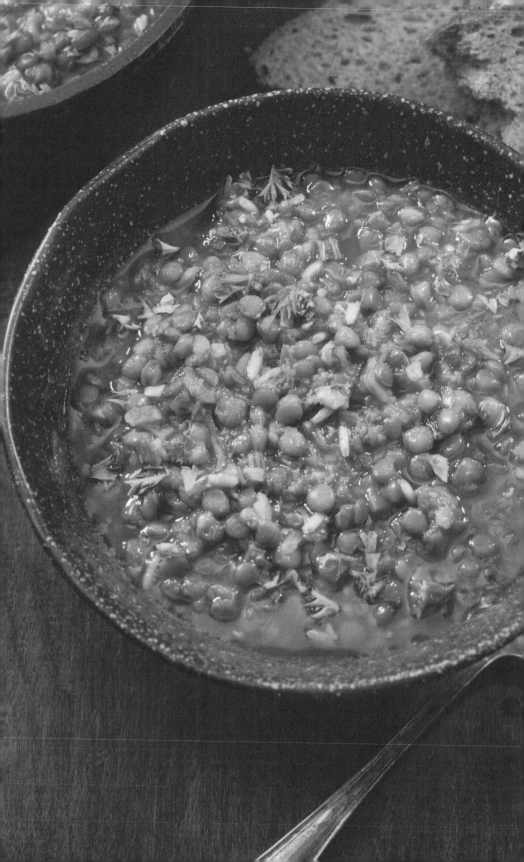

SAVORY RECIPES

Teri's Vitality Stew

1 tbl coconut oil
1 medium onion, minced
1 large carrot, grated
2 stalks celery, chopped
1 cup millet or basmati rice
10-12 cups organic chicken stock
1 cup green or red lentils
3 cloves garlic
1 tbl curry powder
2 tsp cumin
Salt and pepper to taste
1 can coconut milk
5 drops celery seed essential oil

Garnishes: Parmesan cheese, parsley, and liquid aminos soy sauce alternative

In large soup pot, heat coconut oil over medium heat and sauté minced onion, carrots, and celery until soft. Add millet or rice and stir. Add chicken stock, lentils, and seasonings—everything but the coconut milk, celery seed essential oil, and garnishes.

Bring to a boil, lower heat, cover, and simmer for 45 minutes. Add coconut milk. Cover and simmer another 10-15 minutes. Adjust seasonings to taste. Stir in 5 drops celery seed essential oil.

Sprinkle each bowl of Vitality Stew with Parmesan cheese, a little parsley, and a dash of liquid aminos soy sauce alternative (optional). Serves eight.

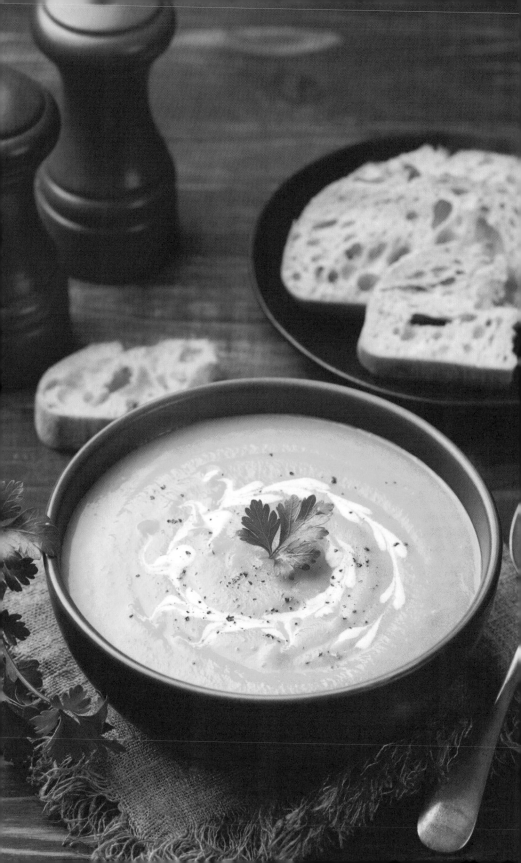

Carrot-Dill Soup

2 tbl unsalted butter
1 onion, coarsely chopped
12 carrots, thinly sliced
5 cups organic chicken stock
1 medium sweet potato, thinly sliced
1 white potato, thinly sliced
1/8 cup fresh dill, minced, or 1 toothpick dipped into dill essential oil
1 tbl fresh lemon juice

Garnishes: sour cream or yogurt; fresh dill

Heat butter in large soup pot and sauté onion over medium heat. Add carrots and chicken stock. Bring to a boil, then turn down to simmer. Add potatoes. Simmer till tender.

Puree soup in blender or food processor in batches. Return to pot. Add fresh dill or dill essential oil and lemon juice and simmer until ready to serve.

To thin, add more stock, milk, cream, or non-dairy milk. Serve hot with a dollop of organic sour cream or yogurt and a sprig of fresh dill. Serves eight.

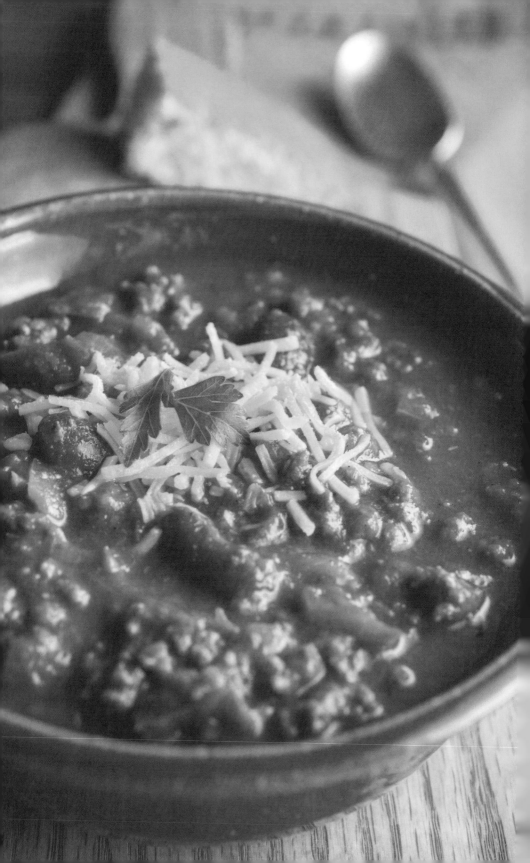

Deluxe Chili

2 tbl olive oil
2 cloves garlic, minced
3 medium onions, minced
2 lb lean ground chuck
2 28-oz cans tomatoes, diced, with juice
1 15-oz can red kidney beans, rinsed and drained (or 2 cups dried
red kidney beans, cooked)
3 cups organic beef broth
1 6-oz can tomato paste
3 tbl chili powder
2 tsp cumin powder
1 to 2 tsp salt to taste
1 toothpick dipped into oregano essential oil
1 toothpick dipped into basil essential oil
Freshly ground pepper

Heat oil in large soup pot. Sauté garlic and onion until translucent. Add meat to soup pot, brown about 10 minutes. Drain off grease. Add tomatoes and juice. Add remaining ingredients, bring to a boil, and then simmer for 1 hour, stirring occasionally. Adjust seasonings to taste. Serves 12. When reheating, thin with beef stock, if needed.

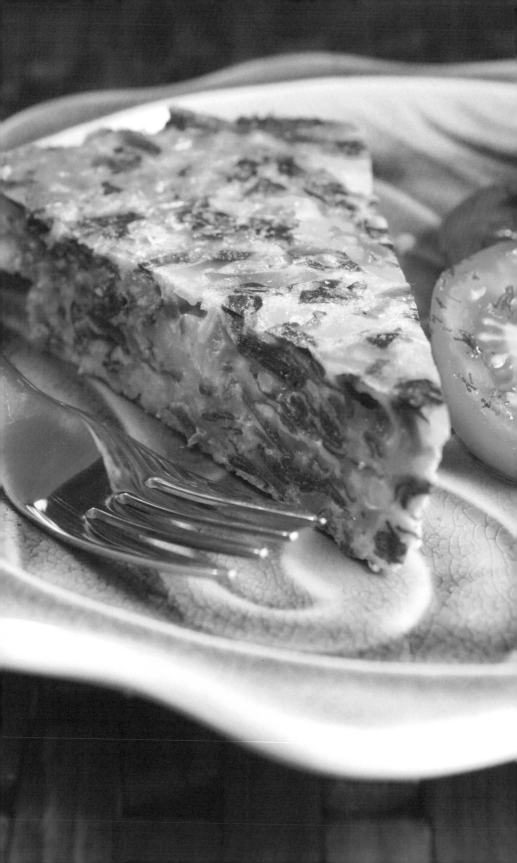

Organic Veggie Pie

Makes one 9-inch pie
1 whole wheat pie crust*
1 cup raw milk Monterey Jack cheese, grated
1 cup raw milk cheddar cheese, grated
3/4 cup spinach or vegetables of your choice, finely chopped
3 large organic eggs
1 cup whole or non-dairy milk
1 tbl whole wheat flour
1 toothpick dipped into nutmeg essential oil
1/4 tsp dry mustard

Preheat oven to 350 degrees F. Fill pie shell with the grated cheese. Top with spinach or vegetables. In a blender, blend eggs, milk, flour, nutmeg essential oil, and mustard together at a low speed for a few seconds. Pour egg mixture into the pie shell.

Bake until eggs are set and lightly brown on top, about 1 hour. If your egg mixture doesn't cover all the vegetables, add more egg mixture or cover with an inverted pie pan so they do not dry out or burn. (I avoid using aluminum foil.)

Variation: Try my family's favorite combinations: yellow squash, red pepper, plus green and yellow onions; broccoli and cauliflower; or whatever you have on hand.

*See *Eating Out of Heaven's Garden* for my Almond Pecan Nut Pie Crust recipe.

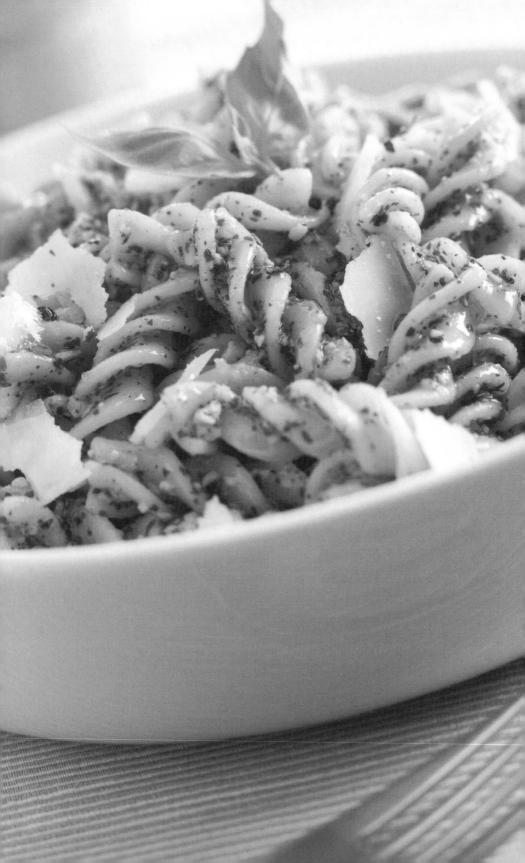

Exquisite Pasta with Pesto & Pine Nuts

1 lb penne pasta, made from durum wheat
Water
Salt
Olive oil
Teri's Famous Pesto Sauce (recipe follows)

Garnishes: sliced tomatoes, raw or toasted pine nuts, and grated Parmesan cheese

Boil salted water in pasta pot. Cook pasta until *al dente*; do not over-cook. Drain and immediately toss with a small amount of olive oil to keep from sticking.

Add pesto sauce to the pasta and toss. Place in warmed serving bowl. Garnish with fresh cut organic tomatoes and sprinkle with Parmesan cheese and pine nuts. Serve with additional grated Parmesan on table.

Variations: Top pasta with bite-sized pieces of sautéed chicken breast before garnishing with Parmesan and pine nuts. Serve with a green salad. Serves four.

Teri's Famous Pesto Sauce

2 cups fresh sweet basil leaves
3/4 cup olive oil
3 cloves garlic
Dash salt
1/2 cup Parmesan cheese, grated

In food processor, blend all ingredients for 1 minute. Set aside until ready to add to pasta.

Keeps well up to three days in refrigerator.

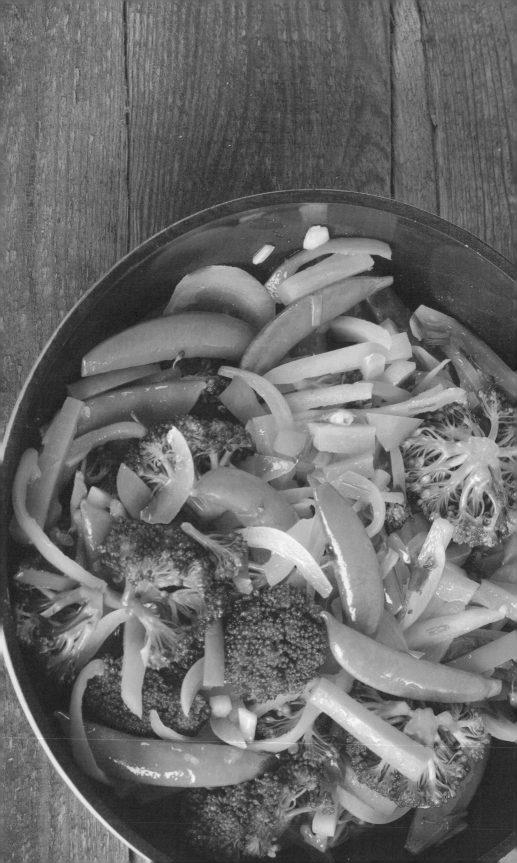

Medley of Stir-Fried Vegetables

1 tbl sesame oil
1 medium onion, chopped
3 carrots, cut diagonally
1/2 head cauliflower, in florets
1 bunch broccoli, in florets
1 cup celery, cut diagonally
3 cloves garlic, minced
1/2 large red bell pepper, cut into strips
1 yellow squash, sliced
1 cup fresh snow peas
1 can water chestnuts, sliced
Mung bean sprouts (optional)

Put sesame oil in your wok or deep frying pan and heat over hot burner. Add onions first. Stirring constantly, add the hardest vegetables first, such as carrots and cauliflower. After 1-2 minutes of stir-frying, add the softer vegetables such as celery, garlic, red bell pepper, and squash. Finally, add the water chestnuts and snow peas, which take just a minute to become tender-crisp.

A nice addition right at the end is a large handful of mung bean sprouts.

Season with my Tangy Stir-Fry Sauce and serve over brown rice.

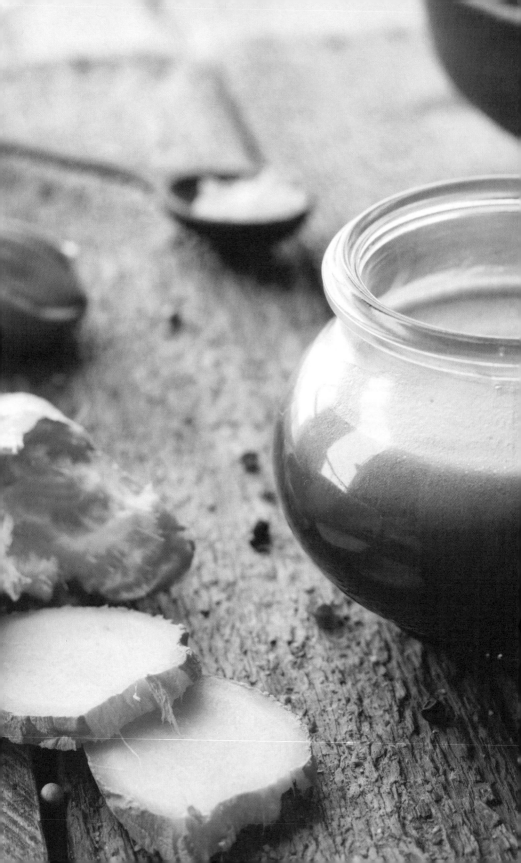

Tangy Stir-Fry Sauce

1/2 cup orange juice
3 drops orange essential oil
1/4 cup liquid aminos soy sauce alternative
1 tbl fresh ginger, grated, plus 1 drop ginger essential oil
2-3 cloves garlic, minced
1-2 tbl raw honey
2 tsp toasted sesame oil
1 tsp arrowroot or 1 tbl cornstarch

Combine everything except the arrowroot or cornstarch. Place the arrowroot or cornstarch in a bowl. Whisk the liquid mixture into it and set aside.

When your stir-fried vegetables are about two-thirds cooked, whisk the liquid mixture again and quickly add it to the wok. Stir from the bottom constantly so all of the vegetables are coated and they won't stick to the bottom.

Turn heat to medium and cook until sauce thickens, just 1-2 minutes. Enjoy!

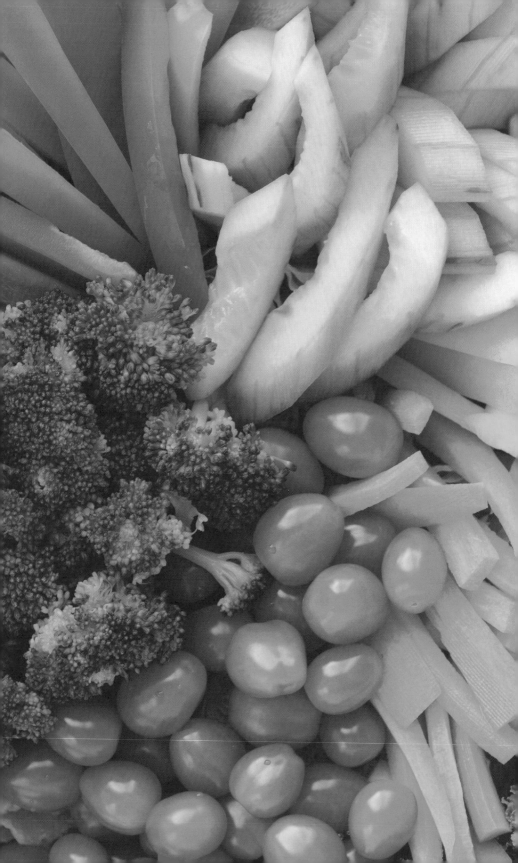

Crudités

1 medium head broccoli
1 pint cherry tomatoes
1/2 lb fresh mushrooms
4 medium cucumbers
1 small bunch radishes
1 1/2 lb carrots
1 large can black olives

Cut broccoli into bite-sized pieces. Steam for 3-5 minutes, drain, and refresh in cold water. Drain thoroughly.

Steam carrots for 3-5 minutes. Drain and refresh in cold water.

Combine all ingredients in a bowl. If desired, pour Crudités Marinade over all, mix gently, and then marinate several hours in the refrigerator. Or serve with Lemon-Garlic Salad Dressing.

Marinade for Crudités

3/4 cup olive oil
1/4 cup red wine vinegar
3 cloves garlic
2 tsp Dijon mustard
2 tsp fresh sweet basil leaves
1 tsp oregano
1 tsp marjoram
1/4 cup parsley, finely minced
1/4 cup chives, finely minced
Salt and pepper to taste

Whisk all ingredients together. Pour over crudités.

Variation: Deepen the marinade's herbal flavor by adding 1/4 drop basil, oregano, and/or marjoram essential oils. Simply dip a clean toothpick into the bottle of essential oil, then stir the toothpick in the marinade.

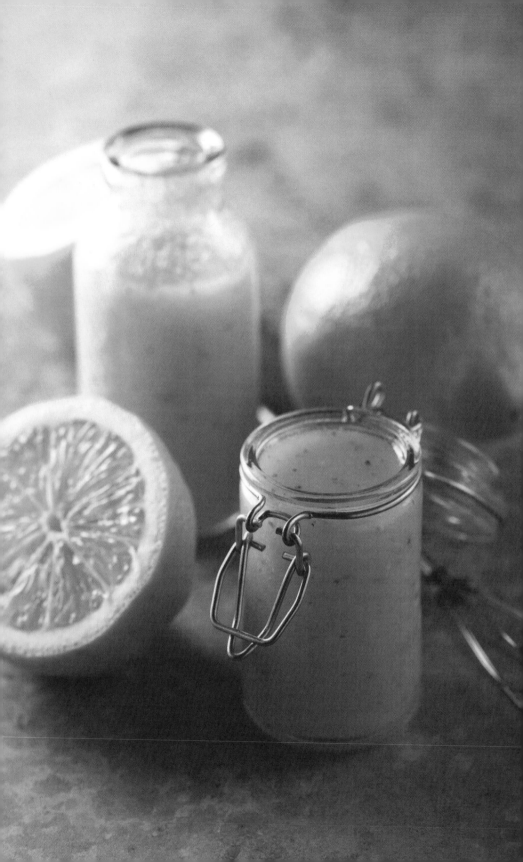

Jeanne's Lemon-Garlic Salad Dressing

Juice of 2 lemons
3 cloves minced garlic
1 1/2 cups organic olive oil
Salt and pepper to taste
3 drops lemon essential oil

Whisk all ingredients thoroughly. Shake before serving.

Baking with Essential Oils

Talk about heaven on earth—wait until you start baking with essential oils! When someone walks into your kitchen and you are baking with essential oils like cinnamon, nutmeg, peppermint, orange, lemon, tangerine, clove, ginger, or lavender, the smell is sure to put a smile on their face!

Sometimes, I put a few drops of these in a warm pot of water and keep the heat on simmer, just to enjoy the aroma!

Any opportunity I have to make organic whipping cream for a recipe, I always flavor it with three or four drops of orange, lemon, or tangerine oil, along with a little bit of agave nectar. You've never had whipping cream like this before!

Because you will be putting your baked goods in the oven, you will lose some of the nutritional benefits of the essential oil. However, you will win every time in flavor and enjoyment.

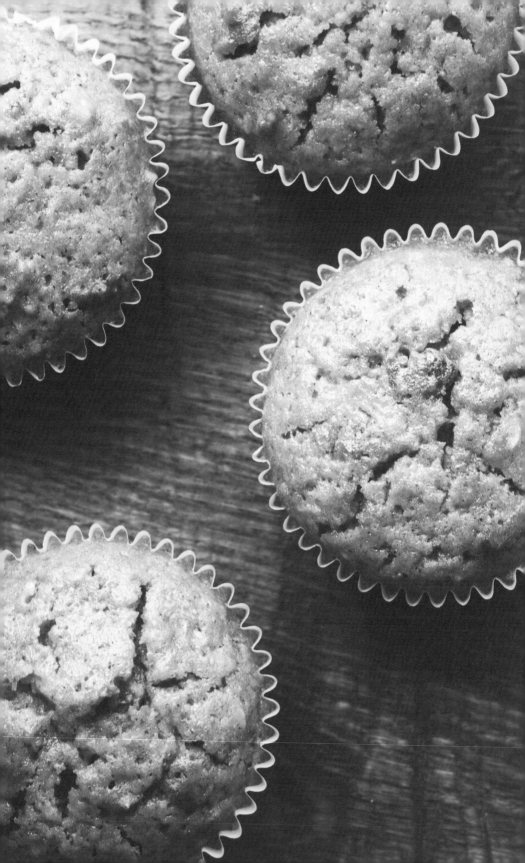

Pumpkin Muffins

Makes 2 dozen
3 1/3 cups whole wheat pastry flour
2 tsp baking soda
1 tsp nutmeg
1/2 tsp allspice
2 tsp salt
2 cups pumpkin puree
2 cups pure maple syrup
4 eggs
1 cup safflower oil
2/3 cup water
1/2 drop cinnamon essential oil
1/2 drop ginger essential oil
1 cup chopped nuts
1/2 cup raisins
2-3 carrots, finely grated

Preheat oven to 375 degrees F. Oil or grease muffin cups.

Sift together flour, baking soda, nutmeg, allspice, and salt.

In a separate bowl, mix wet ingredients well. Stir in essential oils.

Make a "well" in the middle of the dry ingredients and pour all of the wet ingredients into it. Mix well.

Add nuts, raisins, and carrots. Mix well.

Pour batter into muffin cups.

Bake for 15-20 minutes. Delicious served hot with a little real butter on them. Better yet, frost them with my Honey Cream Cheese Frosting recipe.

Tip: Enjoy fresh muffins all week. This batter stores beautifully for several days in the refrigerator. Just scoop out what you need and bake.

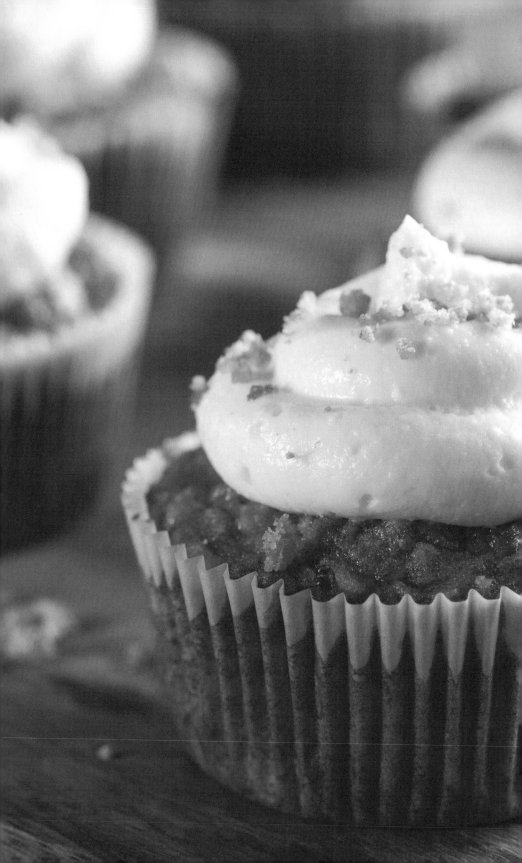

Honey Cream Cheese Frosting

32 oz cream cheese
1/2 cup butter
1 tsp natural vanilla extract
1 cup raw honey (a light-colored honey works best for this frosting)
3-4 drops orange essential oil

Whip all ingredients with a food processor or hand mixer until smooth. (Cream cheese and butter must be softened if you're going to use a hand mixer.)

Spread on cooled pumpkin muffins, cinnamon rolls, or cake just before serving.

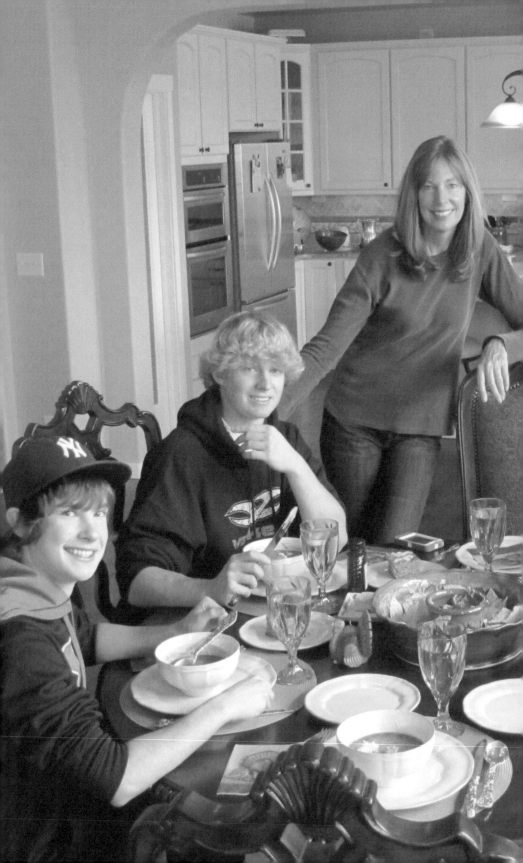

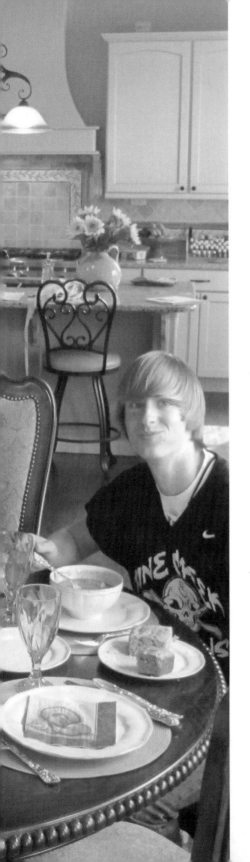

Always Make More Than You Need!

As we conclude our discussion on creative cooking with essential oils, I'd like to share a joyful story to illustrate the tremendous impact any parent can have through the love of food.

When my youngest son, Joseph, was a junior in high school, our family moved from Arizona to Colorado. Thinking about how hard it was to become accustomed to a new school and make friends, I texted him: "Hey Joseph, would you like to invite a couple of guys over for lunch tomorrow? If you met anybody this week, I'd love to cook you all some lunch."

"Sure," he immediately replied.

Score! I thought and off I went to the store. By noon the next day, I had made enough food for an army! Suddenly, not one, but two cars pulled up to the house and out piled seven football players, plus Joseph. Thank goodness my mother always taught us to make more than you think you need.

The lunch was such a success that the following Thursday, Joseph texted me to ask if I could make lunch for the guys again. This went on week after week until the Friday before Christmas, when we had twenty guests for my famous organic pizzas. When I had to be out of town a few times, my amazing sisters, Jan and Jill, came down from Denver just to make this special Friday lunch.

The best part is that these teenagers came to trust me enough to confide in me when they needed a sympathetic ear. Some learned to pray before meals. And this mama's heart felt good knowing her son was acclimating well after our long-distance move.

Ladies, God chose us to be the atmosphere builders in the home. We are the pace-setters, the interior designers. We decide what our families and our guests will see, hear, smell, and taste when they are in our home. This is our privilege.

My prayer is that all of the neighborhood children will want to come to your home. I once read, "Mothers are angels in training." That's you! Receive it, embrace it, and enjoy it!

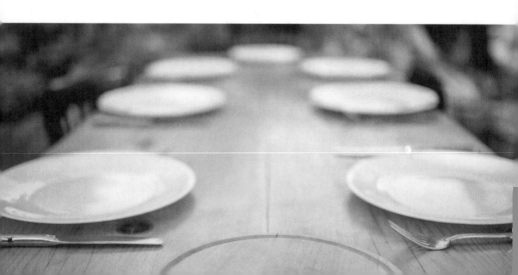

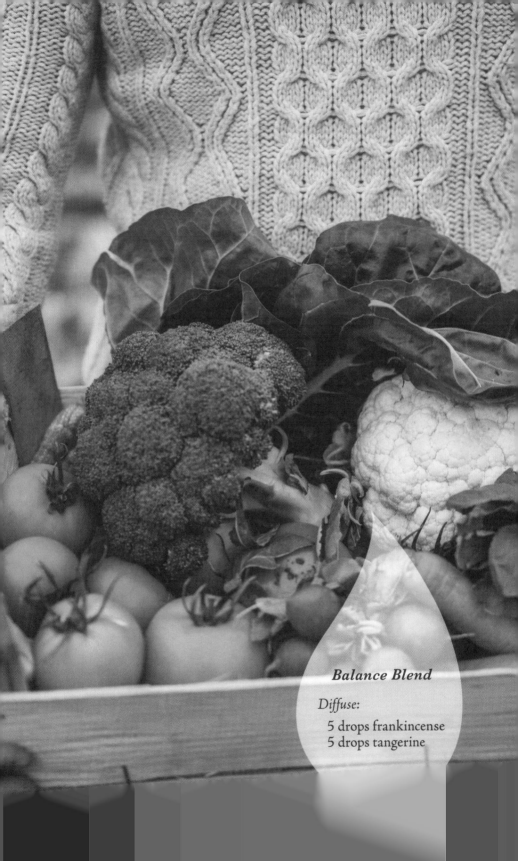

Balance Blend

Diffuse:

5 drops frankincense
5 drops tangerine

UNTIL THE DAY BREAKS AND
THE SHADOWS FLEE AWAY, I WILL GO MY WAY
TO THE MOUNTAIN OF MYRRH AND TO
THE HILL OF FRANKINCENSE.

—SONG OF SOLOMON 4:6 (NKJV)

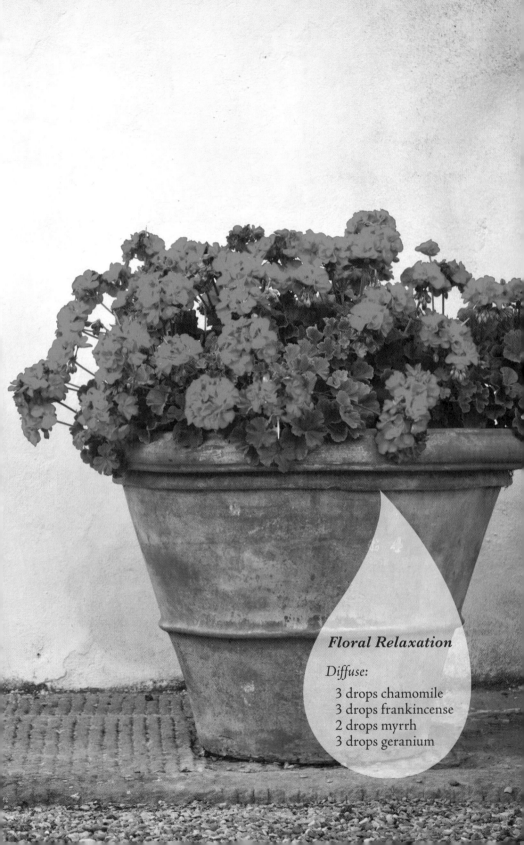

Floral Relaxation

Diffuse:

3 drops chamomile
3 drops frankincense
2 drops myrrh
3 drops geranium

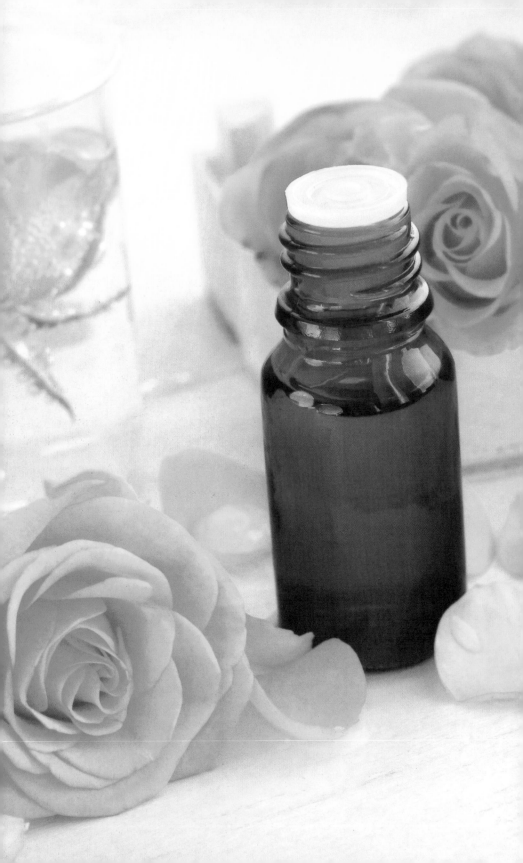

8

ESSENTIAL OILS FOR EXTRAVAGANT ROMANCE

Perfume and incense bring joy to the heart.
—Proverbs 27:9

One of the greatest forces in the universe is, and always will be, the physical intimacy of a couple in love. Wars are fought, nations are conquered, and battles rage over love. The extraordinary way that God created the bodies of men and women shows His tender, creative, and passionate nature.

In the book, *The Act of Marriage: The Beauty of Sexual Love*, authors Tim and Beverly LaHaye say:

Because the Bible clearly and repeatedly speaks out against the misuse or abuse of sex, labeling it "adultery" or "fornication," many people—either innocently or as a means of trying to justify their immorality—have misinterpreted the teaching and concluded that God condemns all sex. However, the contrary is true. The Bible always speaks approvingly of this relationship—as long as it is confined to married partners. The only prohibition on sex in the Scripture relates to extramarital or premarital activity. Without question, the Bible is abundantly clear on that subject, condemning all such conduct. God is the creator of sex. He set our human drives in motion, not to torture men and women, but to bring them enjoyment and fulfillment.[50]

There is so much confusion among people of faith on this subject, evidenced by the millions of dollars spent every year on books that specifically deal with igniting romance in a marriage. I hope that by the end of this chapter, you will feel hopeful, expectant, and enthusiastic.

Being a traditionalist, allow me to add a subtitle to this chapter: "For Married Couples Only." There is an important verse in Scripture instructing us about this: "*I charge you, O daughters of Jerusalem, by the gazelles or by the does of the field, do not stir up nor awaken love until it pleases*" (Song of Solomon 2:7 NKJV). "Until it pleases" means at the appropriate time.

If you're not married, I encourage you to skip this chapter for now. If you are engaged to be married, read with caution and prayerfully consider the preparations you and your future spouse will make to have maximum fulfillment in this part of your marriage.

If you *are* married and wish to have increased pleasure, extravagant romance, and lasting enjoyment in the bedroom, read on.

Smells Trigger Our Emotions

Have you ever pondered why women spend so much money on perfume? Why men often find one cologne they like and use it year after year? It's simple: smell produces thought and thought triggers emotion.

Suppose you walk past a bakery and suddenly, your nose detects the smell of cinnamon wafting through the air. If your grandmother used to bake cinnamon rolls, you might instantly have a happy memory of her triggered by that smell.

Men, if you love to go hunting in the forest or woodlands, there are certain trees so familiar to you that if I put a bottle of spruce, pine, or balsam fir essential oil under your nose, you might immediately think back to one of your hunting trips.

Every essential oil provides both physical support for the body and emotional support for the soul. When it comes to love and physical intimacy, an essential oil can have a positive effect on your hormones (your body) and increase your desire to enjoy intimacy with your spouse (your soul).

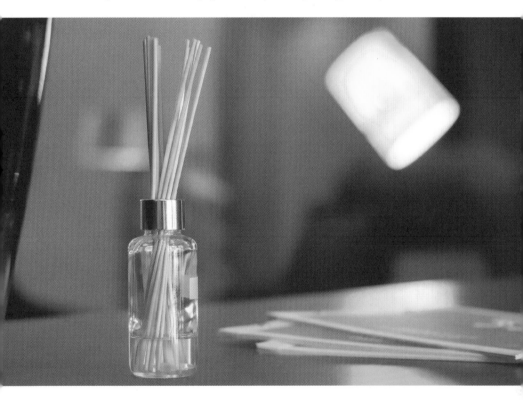

The Power of Scent

One of the funniest things that has ever happened to me perfectly illustrates the power of scent. I was standing in line at the airport, waiting to check in for an international flight. When my turn finally came, I put my bags on the scale and a very stern-looking airline worker looked down at me.

"Are you kidding me?" he exclaimed. "Your bags are so overweight, it is going to cost you $140!"

Everyone stared at me. Without even thinking, I took two steps toward the man, planning to pull out my wallet and hand him my credit card. But that particular day, I was wearing one of my absolute favorite blends of essential oils. Suddenly, the man looked up, took off his glasses, and literally sniffed a couple of times—like he was trying to get a better whiff of my scent! Then he declared, "Actually, for today, I think I can waive your fee."

The chatter around me just ceased and all eyes were on me. I'm sure they were wondering what could have changed this guy's mind. But I knew. And I now wear that scent every time I go to the airport.

In my business as a personal wellness coach, I have a client who once came to me very upset, complaining that her husband was always grumpy and she could not cheer him up no matter what she did.

I asked if her husband would be willing to use some essential oils for his emotions. She said, "Absolutely not!" Thinking outside the box, I said, "That's okay. Let's try something else." I gave her an essential oil to take home and try. I encouraged her to wear it as a perfume and intentionally try to get really close to her husband wherever he was in the house so he could smell it. I even had her put a drop in his shoes at night.

She called me a few days later and said, "By golly, it worked!" His attitude had improved without him realizing what was going on.

Scent has a powerful way of changing our outlook. If the sizzle has gone out of your marriage, don't despair. There's always an essential oil available to help every situation. Before we dive into oils for romance, however, let's address a couple of touchy subjects first.

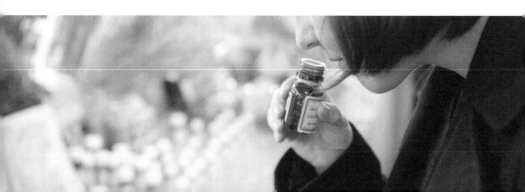

Love vs. Lust

There is a vast difference between love and lust. Love cherishes, protects, and heals. Love is unselfish, cares about the pleasure of another, holds no grudges, leaves the past behind, and embraces the future. Love forgives. *"Love bears all things, believes all things, hopes all things, endures all things"* (1 Corinthians 13:7 ESV). In other words, love is from God. In fact, *"God is love"* (1 John 4:8).

On the other hand, lust is self-absorbed, jealous, and demanding. Lust pushes another person, no matter what they want or need. Lust is short-sighted and leaves you empty. Lust is of the flesh, with no emotions involved. God's Word tells us, *"The mind governed by the flesh is death"* (Romans 8:6).

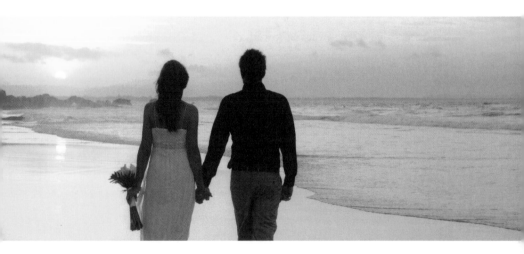

Loving Well

A great physical relationship with your spouse begins with a decision to love well. That decision needs to be firmly planted in your mind and then your heart will carry it out on a daily basis.

When past disappointments are forgiven and respect is restored, you can embark on a journey you never imagined was possible. This journey includes the exciting physical relationship that God desires for your marriage.

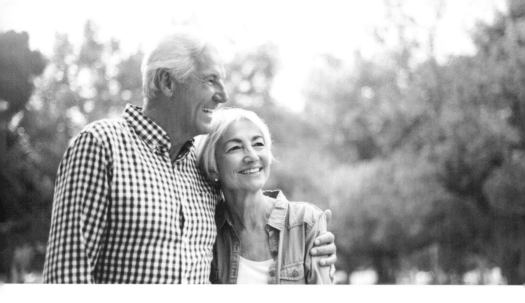

Cherishing Each Other

If you are not in a good place in your marriage, I highly recommend that you read *Cherish: The One Word That Changes Everything for Your Marriage* by Gary Thomas. It's the best book I've read on marriage in twenty years.

Most of us were never mentored in this area of cherishing one another. Being in a place of mutual love and respect is crucial before trying to fix the physical part of marriage. As Thomas explains in his book:

> The way we treat something acknowledges whether we cherish it or hold it with indifference or contempt. To truly cherish something is to go out of our way to show it off, protect it, and honor it.... God can give us hearts to delight in each other so we can enjoy a marriage where we sometimes even feel guilty because we have it so good. Most of us don't want marriages where we grit our teeth and tolerate each other just because God's Word says we don't "qualify" for a divorce. Most of us don't want marriages where our spouses really don't like us, much less respect us. We want to be cherished, and we want to be married to someone we cherish.[51]

Making Time for Pleasure

The use of essential oils for romance oozes out of the pages of Song of Songs, Proverbs, and the Psalms. In the Scriptures, we see oils poured on people's beds, and liberally used on their clothes. Today, our lives seem so incredibly busy that love can get taken off the front burner and moved to the back one, where it's placed on a slow simmer.

If you're a stay-at-home parent, especially with small children, it can be tough to feel sexy. Nothing is less of a turn-on than a glue stick stuck in one child's hair, another wrapped around your legs pleading for attention, and a crying baby, too. It's easy to prefer a shower and a chance to unwind rather than hot times with your spouse.

It can be just as tough for those working outside the home. After a long day in the office, especially a stressful one, wrapping up in a cozy blanket and watching a movie can seem more appealing than a night of romance.

But we must take time for each other if we don't want our marriages to grow cold and stale because of life circumstances. Men, your woman longs to be the object of your desire. Women, your man longs to be the sexy stud of your dreams and the guy you daydream about.

When married couples come together in passion, it creates contentment and happiness, and builds solidarity and trust. Then there's the bottom line: it's just plain fun and enjoyable.

You're married! Your bedroom should be a place of intimate adoration, not a place to fall asleep while watching television or reading. It's time to put the boom back in the bedroom.

You're Number One

Let's get a little selfish for a minute. If you are the reluctant bedroom partner, think about why that might be. Are you tired or stressed? Do you just not feel like it? All of these things are understandable. Life comes in seasons. Sometimes, we feel full of passion; other times, we feel like a dud. The problem with the dud times is that our spouse can be adversely affected by our reluctance to accept their passionate advances.

Now, before you think I'm here to lecture you about "submitting to the marital act" with one finger wagging at you and my other hand clutching a Bible, let me reassure you, that is *not* my heart. I understand about the dud times—I can totally relate. In fact, when we're just not feeling it but "take one for the team" anyway, that hurts our spouse.

Instead, let's explore what you may be able to do to get yourself in the mood, ignite your passion, and get excited about intimacy again.

If *you* are the willing one and your spouse is the one holding back, hang in there. We are going to go over some tips to help rev your spouse's engine.

Getting Excited About Romance

Ylang Ylang

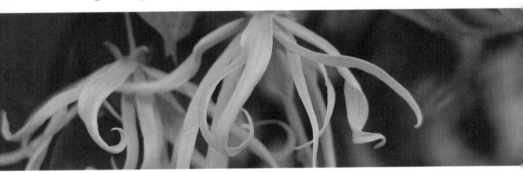

Ylang ylang means "flower of flowers." Traditionally, ylang ylang blossoms have been used to cover the beds of newlywed couples on their wedding nights. Their fragrance is said to bring feelings of calm for both men and women, promote relaxation, and restore confidence. Ylang ylang oil is one of the top ingredients in several perfumes, including Chanel No. 5. Place two to three drops of ylang ylang essential oil on your wrists and neck during the day.

Jasmine

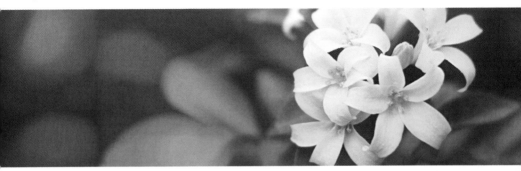

For centuries, women have treasured jasmine for its beautiful, seductive fragrance. With a scent that is uplifting, jasmine can ignite your passion and soothe any feelings that may be blocking your desire for romance. Nicknamed the "queen of night," jasmine flowers must be picked at night to maximize their fragrance; otherwise, the delicate scent will evaporate by sunrise.

Jasmine is actually an "absolute" and not an essential oil. This means the essence of the jasmine flowers is captured using solvent extraction instead of steam distillation. This important difference means that jasmine should not be taken internally. Wear as a perfume or diffuse ten to twenty drops in your bedroom for twenty minutes to an hour.

Rose

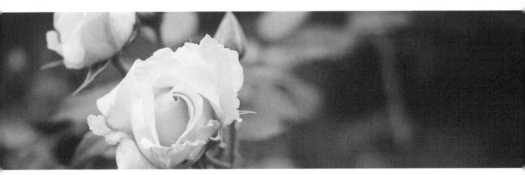

Rose has a beautiful, intoxicating fragrance that creates a sense of well-being and comfort. The rose has long been considered the flower of love and passion, so it's no wonder that this essential oil can help a married couple find joy in the bedroom.

Place five to ten drops of rose essential oil into a cold water diffuser and diffuse for twenty minutes to an hour every day. To use as a perfume, dilute rose essential oil in an unscented carrier oil. Or for a luxurious bath, place five drops of rose essential oil into the bottom of your tub, fill it with warm water, and soak for at least twenty minutes.

Sandalwood

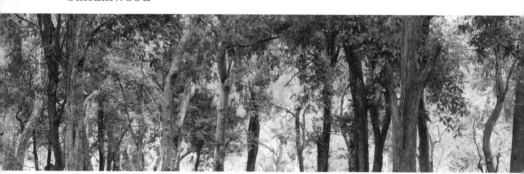

Sandalwood is the most potent natural aphrodisiac in our essential oil arsenal, increasing libido and sexual response. Because it's similar to a man's natural body scent, it sends out a highly effective erotic signal to a woman, even when it's barely perceptible. Sandalwood is high in sesquiterpenes—chemical compounds that stimulate the pineal gland and the limbic part of the brain. The pineal gland is responsible for releasing melatonin, a powerful immune stimulant.

Men can replace their cologne with sandalwood essential oil, placing two drops on the wrists and giving a gentle pat over the face after shaving. Women can diffuse sandalwood to awaken their desire.

Black Pepper

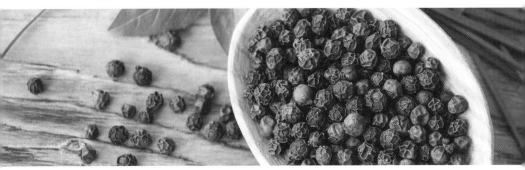

The essential oil of black pepper may sound like an odd choice for romance…but it's hot and spicy, the way we like our love life, right? All joking aside, black pepper is stimulating, energizing, and empowering. A 2002 study in Japan showed that inhaling black pepper oil caused an increase in plasma adrenaline concentration.[52] Simply put, it gets your blood pumping in all the right ways.

Add three to five drops of black pepper essential oil and another favorite essential oil to your diffuser for twenty to sixty minutes.

Ginger

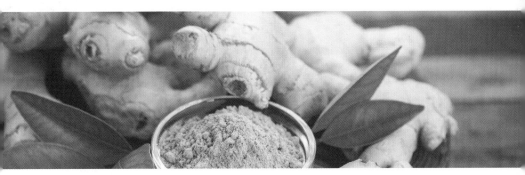

Ginger has a warm fragrance that is gentle yet stimulating; it encourages physical energy and confidence. Women in the West African country of Senegal weave belts of ginger root to restore their mate's sexual potency. Profoundly romantic, refreshing, and arousing, ginger oil can amplify excitement and new heights of intimacy.

Place two drops on the bottom of your feet and around your ankles on a night you are ready for romance. Allow the warming sensation of ginger to awaken desire.

Get the Home Fires Burning

Now, let's address inspiring romance in your spouse. Before we get started, please keep in mind that essential oils cannot be used as tools for manipulation. There is no secret love potion that will instantly turn your bedroom into a nightly romantic getaway for two, make an unwilling spouse leap into bed with you, or force-fix a broken marriage. However, there *are* things we can do to heighten romance and intimacy.

The essential oils that follow are said to inspire genuine love and passion. We recommend wearing these oils in place of cologne or perfume as well as diffusing them in your home.

Geranium

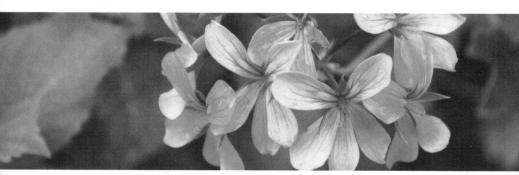

The delightfully floral scent of geranium can soothe anxiety and inspire emotional balance, which opens the heart to romance. Entering a room scented with geranium is uplifting. It makes you want to leave your cares at the door and relax. Geranium can also support the female reproductive system when rubbed on the lower abdomen.

Rosewood

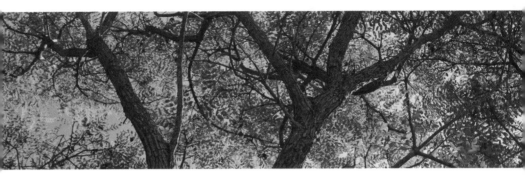

Rosewood essential oil will help to chase away a bad day. It has a calming, light floral scent with a woodsy undertone, creating a feeling of peace and a sense of wholeness. If you or your spouse struggle with intimacy due to stress and workload, this is the essential oil for you.

Vanilla and Lime

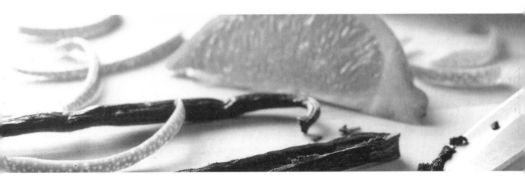

Combining lime and vanilla essential oils delivers an amazing one-two punch! Vanilla is a warming scent that dissolves negative emotions and lowers inhibition. It has been long known as an inviting, sensual scent. Lime essential oil is invigorating and inspires lighthearted emotions. Used together, these oils can inspire playful, romantic notions.

Place five to ten drops of each essential oil into a cold air diffuser and begin diffusing twenty minutes before your spouse arrives home. Continue diffusing for up to forty minutes afterward.

Isn't It Romantic?

Romance can sometimes happen naturally, but for many, this is a skill that must be practiced. Make a habit of being more thoughtful and build up the excitement for your spouse. Creating the environment for a romantic encounter is an art.

> *Let him kiss me with the kisses of his mouth—for your love is more delightful than wine. Pleasing is the fragrance of your perfumes; your name is like perfume poured out. No wonder the young women love you!* (Song of Songs 1:2–3)

It's time to *be* more romantic if you are looking for more romance. Choose oils from the above section and began diffusing and wearing them daily.

If your bedroom is filled with clutter, it's time for a change. Be thoughtful and intentional about your romantic space. Turn off the television and turn on some tender or sensual music. Candlelight is a must, with the added bonus that it makes us look attractive at any age. For an alluring atmosphere, diffuse essential oils into your bedroom about twenty minutes before the passion begins.

Women, if you have been running around all day and you'd like to get in the mood, choose your favorite oil. Rub it on your neck, your wrists, and on your inner thigh area.

Men, if you have had a busy and stressful day, but know you have a date with your wife tonight, sandalwood is your oil. Place it on your wrist and neck. Put two drops on the palms of your hands and breathe deeply for five minutes before entering your home. This will get your mind, body, and emotions in line with your intention.

And if you have never read King Solomon's Song of Songs in bed with your spouse, you are missing out on one of the most alluring things you can do as a couple. It's an exciting book filled with love, romance, longing, and desire. Express these feelings toward each other—and have a little fun as a couple!

How About Massage?

Starting a romantic evening with a massage can be delightful for a number of reasons. First, it builds desire. Second, there is no instant gratification. You must wait while you serve your spouse. When each person feels cherished, your physical body naturally responds better.

Open up each romantic essential oil and breathe in the fragrances together. You can choose one oil together or one for each of you. A great combination of essential oils is rose and geranium. Or try ylang ylang for women and Idaho balsam fir for men.

Place five drops of your chosen oil into coconut oil and mix. You can also apply a few drops of the oil down your spouse's spine before you give them an indulgent massage. The spine has nerve endings that efficiently transport the oils to the entire body. If your intention is truly to give rather than receive, this will be a very loving experience.

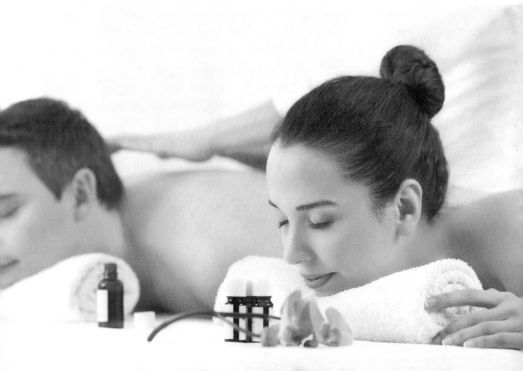

Special Romantic Oils for Men

His cheeks are as a bed of spices, as sweet flowers: his lips like lilies, dropping sweet smelling myrrh. (Song of Solomon 5:13 KJV)

Men, if you are reluctant to follow your spouse into the world of essential oils for romance, read the above Scripture verse. The woman in the Song of Solomon is speaking about her beloved. *He* is like a bed of spices and sweet flowers. *He* is dripping with sweet-smelling myrrh. This sounds like a man who loves to get romantic.

Here are some exciting oils just for men that can help you enhance and inspire your romantic life. (You can also review chapter 6 to learn more about balancing your hormones and specific struggles men can have.)

Overall Romance

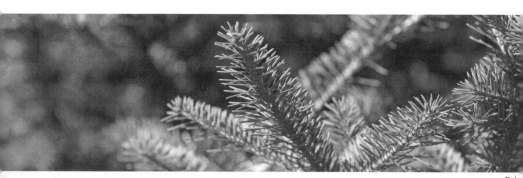

Balsa

Balsam fir essential oil has a woodsy, manly smell that will take your mind right to the forest. Both men and women find its scent to be grounding, balancing, relaxing to the body, and stimulating to the mind.

This is a favorite men's cologne for many of our circle of male friends. I constantly have wives thanking me for sharing the information with them about this oil. While a husband may fantasize about intimacy with his wife in the forest, she is happy to be enjoying the whole experience in the comfort of their bedroom...without the mosquitos!

Erectile Dysfunction

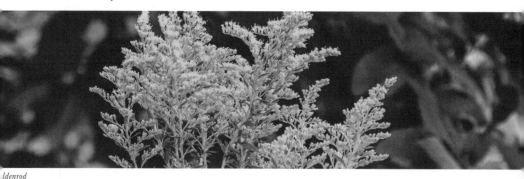

ldenrod

Essential oil of goldenrod is very helpful for erectile dysfunction because it helps to improve blood flow in the body, which benefits manly function. Ironically, the Pilgrims named goldenrod "Liberty Tea!"

Rub a few drops of goldenrod on the soles of the feet and then dilute with olive oil and apply close to (not on) your private parts each night before bed.

Low Sex Drive in Men

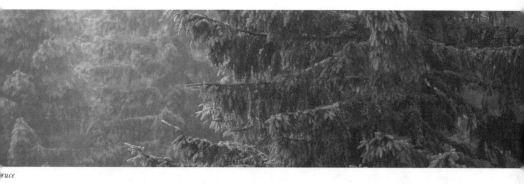

ruce

Two really good essential oils for low sex drive are sandalwood and spruce. These oils will help to raise a man's testosterone levels naturally, with no side effects. Take five to eight drops of each and rub on the bottoms of your feet each night before bed.

In a glass jar, mix two ounces of olive oil, ten drops of sandalwood, and ten drops of spruce. Right before intimacy with your wife, rub this mixture on your lower abdomen and inner thighs. Be sure to keep the jar in a safe place and use as needed.

Boost Confidence and Testosterone

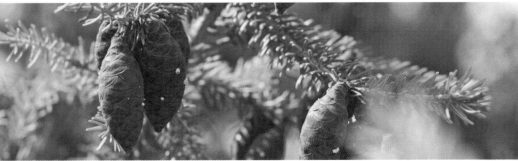

Black Spruce

Northern lights black spruce essential oil increases testosterone levels and confidence in a man. It's a very appealing when applied like a cologne or an aftershave. Women are drawn to a man wearing this scent. It is similar to balsam fir in that it transports your mind right to a lush forest.

Romantic Oils for Women

Ylang ylang, mentioned previously, is one of the most glorious, romantic oils for women. There are several others that are wonderful to use to increase romance.

Clary Sage

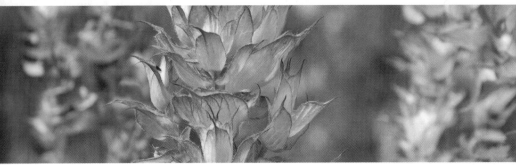

Clary Sage

Ever wonder why women may feel friskier at certain times and not so much at other times? When a woman is ovulating, her estrogen levels are naturally higher. God designed women to feel more "in the mood" when they are fertile. As women age, their estrogen levels decrease.

One sign of a low estrogen level is vaginal dryness. Using a drop of clary sage daily can help to raise the estrogen level and combat this problem.

While there are many synthetic estrogen products on the market, I do not recommend them, as they can have potentially harmful side effects. God gave us every tree, plant, flower, and shrub on the third day of creation to use as our medicine. And *their* side effects are marvelous.

For the best results, apply clary sage on your forearms, wrists, back of the neck, or below the navel.

Rose

If you are looking to bring excitement back to your marriage, try rose essential oil. This intoxicating and alluring scent awakens sleeping desire and stirs longing. It's no wonder that rose is considered the flower of love. Wear rose essential oil as a perfume and enjoy.

Jasmine

For centuries, jasmine has been known for its beautiful and seductive fragrance. The scent is known to increase libido, getting you in the mood for love and romance. This delightful scent naturally releases serotonin in the brain and helps to relieve depression.

Romantic Oils for Both of You

Healthy Blood Flow

A healthy blood flow and good circulation are keys to satisfying intimacy. Cypress essential oil is helpful for both men and women when rubbed on the inner thighs.

Women can try mixing it with ylang ylang or clary sage. Men can mix cypress with a favorite manly oil like sandalwood or balsam fir.

For Nervous Newlyweds

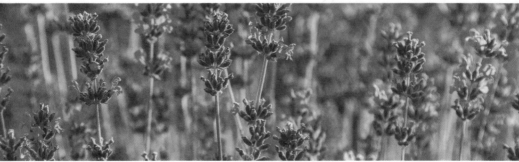

Lavend

Are you soon-to-be married and feeling nervous about the wedding night and the honeymoon? Try mixing fifteen drops of lavender essential oil with four ounces of coconut oil in a glass container. Apply topically during a sensual massage for relaxation. You can also breathe in the lavender oil undiluted for an additional feeling of refreshment and ease.

Orange You Glad…

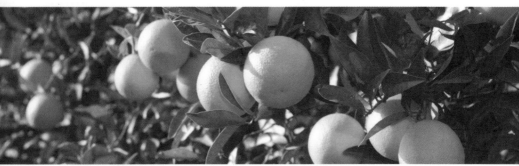

Orar

John Lennon reportedly once said he wanted a song to sound "refreshing and zesty and thirst-quenching—you know, like an orange." While it's not clear what song he was referring to, orange *is* a very happy-smelling essential oil that helps spouses let go of stress and embrace being in the moment. It's a natural aphrodisiac that brightens the mood, lifts the spirits, and promotes carefree intimacy. Diffuse it or mix it with clary sage, cypress, or ylang ylang and apply to your inner thighs.

God's Wonderful Gifts

Are you beginning to see God's extravagant provision for you in romance? In marriage, we must nurture friendship along with physical intimacy. Each is a great treasure and we get to treat them with great care.

As one of the most glorious gifts God has given us, physical intimacy must be handled with extreme tenderness and care. You and your spouse are God's treasured children. We are not each other's property. Remember all of the things that originally attracted you to your spouse, hold them in your heart, and think of them often. It may take a lifetime to truly learn to love your spouse well, but as you enjoy intimacy with one another, your marriage will grow stronger and better.

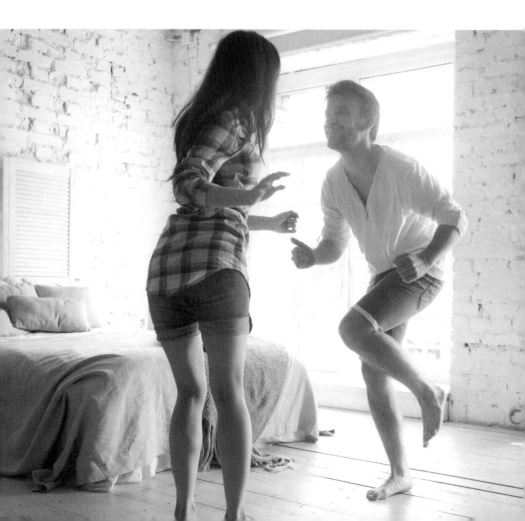

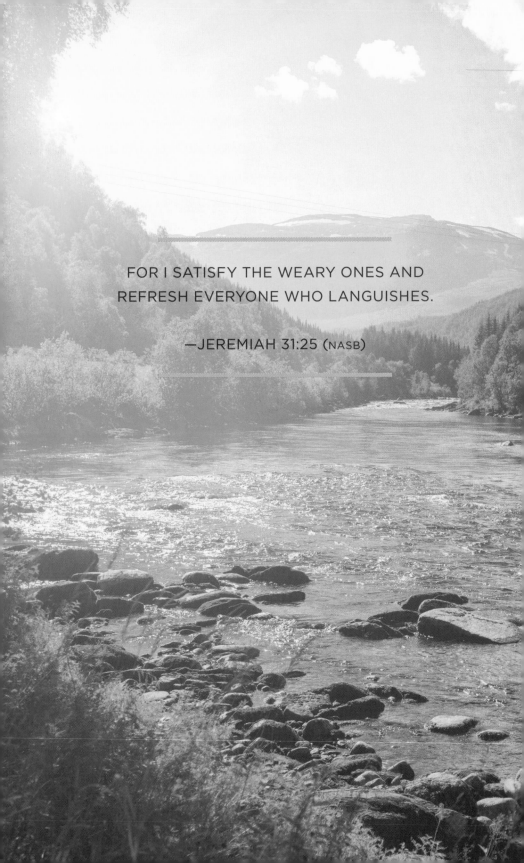

FOR I SATISFY THE WEARY ONES AND
REFRESH EVERYONE WHO LANGUISHES.

—JEREMIAH 31:25 (NASB)

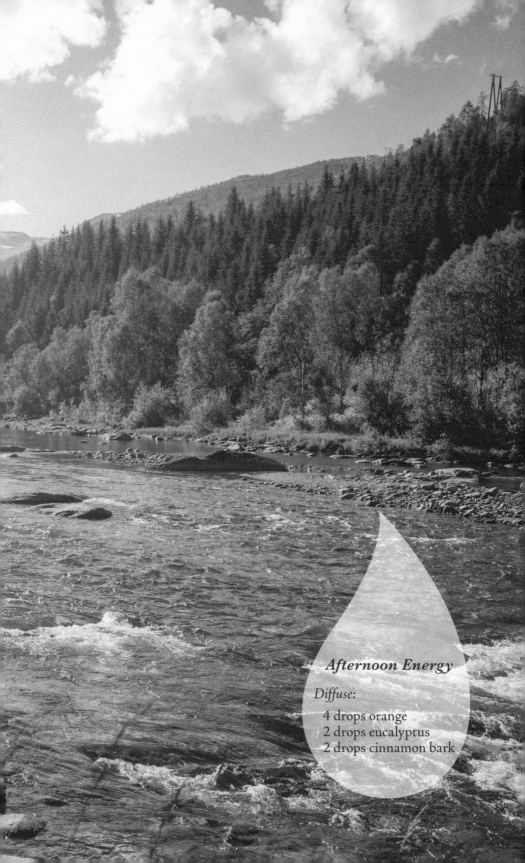

Afternoon Energy

Diffuse:

4 drops orange
2 drops eucalyptus
2 drops cinnamon bark

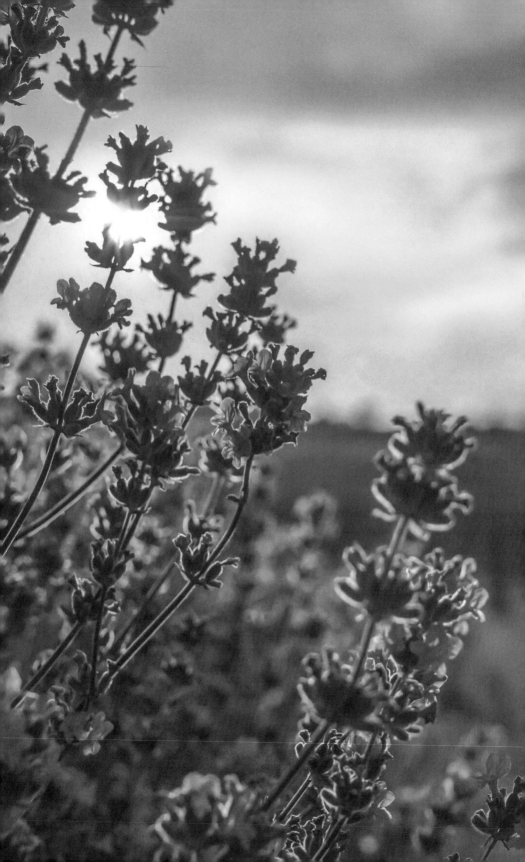

9

RECIPE FOR A JOY-FILLED LIFE

I hope that by now, you are seeing God's heart for you to be truly healthy in your body, your soul, and your spirit. He longs for you to enjoy your life, to wake up with hope in your heart and rest with peace in your mind.

To really see the extravagance of God's provision for our health, let's dig deeper into the subject of *therapeuo* healing that I spoke about in chapter 3. You may recall that *therapeuo* means "healing gradually over time with care and nursing." If you have already been prayed over for a particular health concern, but you have not seen the full fruit of those prayers yet, think about how you can be an active participant in the healing you desire.

Oils work optimally when they are used in support of an overall healthy lifestyle. Whether your struggle is physical, mental, or emotional, you can partner with God for your own therapeuo healing by taking responsibility to nurture and care for yourself at each of these levels. No matter how extravagant God's provision, we still need to do our part to regain vitality. Every journey consists of three things: the things we leave behind; the things we take with us; and the route we follow. The route I am inviting you to follow is a natural one designed by our Creator for maximum vibrant health. Let's leave behind any unhealthy attitudes and habits that would hinder our progress on this ancient path. Let's look at some things we need to take with us in order to reach our goal of living well.

My passion and heart's desire is that you become a secure, vibrant, and healthy person. What follows are some simple, easily accessible things you can do to change your life now.

Take a Walk

Walking is good for every system of your body. If you go on a fast power walk—if your doctor says it's okay, of course—you are getting your heart muscle working and oxygenating your brain. You can wake up in a total slump, yet once you start walking, you will suddenly feel better emotionally. One of the top causes of depression is a lack of oxygen in the brain and walking gives it a free mini-vacation.

A couple of years ago, I taught an all-day seminar with Patricia King on the subject of health. In one of our sessions, I shared my passion for walking. It's a known fact that President Abraham Lincoln made some of his most important decisions while taking his daily walk. In the Scriptures, we see that Adam walked, Abraham walked, and Moses walked—we were born to be walkers!

Well, there was a man sitting in the back of the room at this seminar who did not seem to be particularly inspired. Even so, he went home…and something came over him. His spirit man rose up and he knew it was time to make some positive changes. He called me eight months later.

"Teri, remember me sitting in the back at your seminar in Arizona?" he said excitedly. "I want you to know I have lost forty pounds and it has changed my life!"

I was so proud of him! I asked him to tell me about all of the dietary changes he had made.

"Oh, no, I have not changed anything in my diet," he said. "I just started walking."

Imagine that—this man lost five pounds a month just by walking.

Friend, this can be you too! If you just start power walking three times a week for twenty minutes a day and work your way up to forty-five minutes a day, five to six times a week, you will see some great changes in the way you feel and you have the potential to release some significant weight. It's easy to add a few more steps to each day by parking your car further away from your destination or taking the stairs instead of the elevator every chance you get.

My final tip is this: when you get home from your walk, instead of getting into the shower and rushing off to work or appointments, take just ten minutes and lie down on the couch or on your carpet and put your feet up. Put about three drops of lemon essential oil in a ten-ounce glass of water and sip it while you are resting. The lemon essential oil will help to keep your liver clean and the time you are lying down will rejuvenate you. Now you will have more energy than you ever imagined throughout the remainder of your day.

It's fun to have a walking buddy—and it's helpful to have some support and accountability—but don't let it stop you if you don't have one. Walking gives you time to think, daydream, and notice the natural beauty around you. Personally, some of my best business ideas have come to me while on my morning walk. Walking is an intentional way to begin confronting those unwanted pounds and telling them where to go. So, friend, let's get walking!

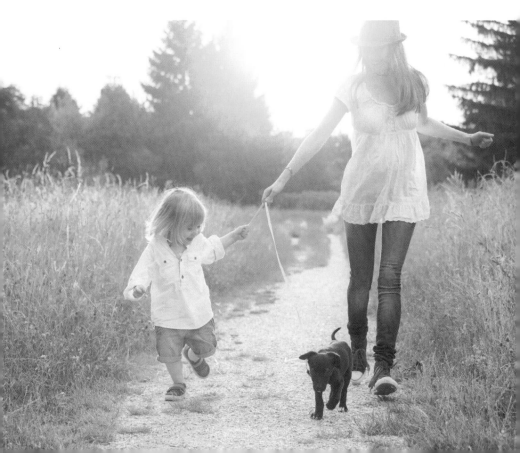

Make Healthy Eating a Celebration

As we discussed in chapter 7, make an intentional choice to eat more "live" foods and be mindful of the source of your foods.

If you don't enjoy cooking, try making it a happy part of your day. Involve your children, spouse, or friends in the cooking process and make it a celebration. Turn on music, sip on a delicious beverage, and dance! Focus on the table setting if that is exciting for you. Add candles, fancy or fun napkins, and special dinner ware. You might approach a family member or friend and take some healthy cooking classes together. Since we all eat three meals a day, why not thoroughly enjoy the experience?

Here are some other tips I've learned:

+ Fall in love with the idea of having meals together as a family.

+ Surrender your cell phones during meal times.

+ Make it an adventure! Add exciting new foods you haven't tried before.

+ If your goal is to improve your nutrition, start by increasing your healthy foods by only 10 percent.

+ Remember to read labels and avoid packaged products that contain ingredients you cannot pronounce.

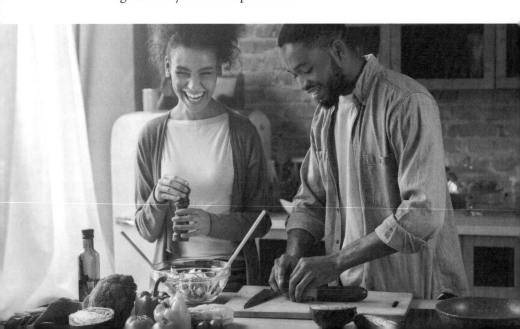

+ Think about starting a "cook or clean" policy. Whoever cooks gets out of kitchen duty!

Food and Essential Oils for Your Mind

To be successful in business and life, you need to have a strong brain and a good mind. There are so many things we can do with food and essential oils to nurture our mind, regardless of our age or season of life. The best brain foods increase alertness and attention span while helping you process new information. Although this is not an exhaustive list, here are a few foods to get you started:

+ High-quality fish like salmon contain omega 3 fatty acids, which reduce brain fog and increase memory and concentration.

+ Walnuts, which actually *look* like your brain, increase memory, alertness, and concentration.

+ Beets increase blood flow to the brain, promoting clear thinking and an increased attention span.

+ Blueberries are high in antioxidants and protect the brain from degeneration, toxins, and stress.

+ Cold-pressed coconut oil and avocado oil support the brain with healthy fats.

These foods increase focus, making them great food options when studying for a big test or preparing for an important meeting.

Here are some essential oils that will give your brain a boost:

+ Cedarwood is useful in helping your brain learn new things. Place one drop of supplement-grade cedarwood essential oil on your thumb and press it to the roof of your mouth before taking on a new project or learning a new subject.

+ Rosemary essential oil has been shown to increase memory and cognitive function while also producing a feeling of contentment. Diffuse rosemary for at least twenty minutes to feel these amazing benefits.

- ✦ Peppermint stimulates the hippocampus area of the brain, which controls mental clarity, focus, and memory.

- ✦ Blue cypress helps your "busy brain." Its soothing properties can help to calm the mind at the end of the day.

By becoming very intentional in your food choices and adding essential oils for your brain, you can nearly stop the aging process in its tracks.

Laughter IS the Best Medicine

When my children were little, we had an animal book about manners. It was so funny that every time I read it to them at bedtime, we all roared. Recently, my daughter found the book in one of her boxes and just the thought of it made us laugh uncontrollably again.

When was the last time you had a really big belly laugh? How long has it been since you and your family or loved ones laughed together? Laughter IS the best medicine.

Years ago, I read about American journalist Norman Cousins, who had a rare disease and was told he only had a few months to live. Cousins didn't want to die in a hospital, so he checked himself out and checked into a hotel. There, he spent hours every day watching comedy movies and TV shows, laughing until his stomach hurt. He lived for another twenty-six years.[53]

Can anyone prove that laughter prolonged Cousins' life? No, but we *do* know that laughter strengthens the immune system, which fights disease.

The Gesundheit! Institute, founded by a medical doctor who clowns, operates under the premise that laughter, joy, and creativity are an integral part of the healing process.[54] God's Word tells us, *"A cheerful heart is good medicine"* (Proverbs 17:22).

I would like to propose a laugh challenge: take the next seven days and watch nothing but funny movies and listen to funny podcasts and uplifting, fun music. Take some notes the day before you start and document how you're feeling during the challenge. Pay attention to your mental state and how your environment changes. How do the people in your life respond?

You may even find that the topics of your conversations change. Pull out your joke books and get started! Connect with me on social media and let me know how it goes.

God loves humor—consider the porcupine, the duckbill platypus, or the big-eyed lemur, not to mention the courtship rituals of many birds. We thrive in places charged with laughter and positivity, too.

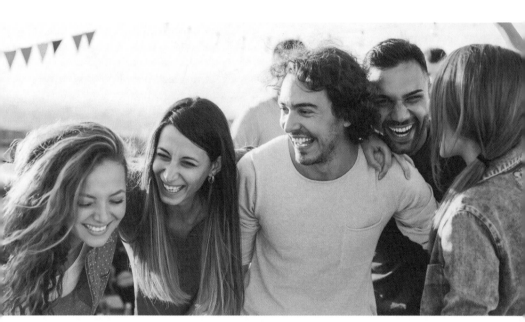

Relationships Bring Joy

A good friend of mine recently said something I think is absolutely brilliant. She said, "I'll know how well I have lived my life by how many people come to my seventieth birthday party." That thought is profound because studies have shown that a life well lived is a life rich with relationships.

Many of us learn very little in school in terms of relating well to other people. We may shy away from making new connections and forging relationships even though this is a key factor to our long-term happiness.

Breathing essential oils can help us find the courage to overcome our anxiety about social interaction. Essential oils that are high in sesquiterpenes have the ability to cross over the blood-brain barrier and release anxiety. Imagine going into a social situation with grace and ease, able to strike up conversations with people you've just met. Start by breathing sandalwood, cedarwood, or frankincense.

If your family has entered into a season of dull routine, I highly recommend turning on a diffuser. Diffusing essential oils in your home can ignite excitement and encourage positive interaction. Studies have shown that diffusing citrus essential oils such as lemon, orange, lime, and tangerine uplift the emotions and release stress. Creating this kind of positive atmosphere in your home can have major benefits for your family.

If it's a romantic relationship you are looking to spark, be sure to read chapter 8.

Your Emotions Matter

Like many people, I have been through some tough times in life. I don't know if we can get all the way through life without some gut-wrenching situations that totally derail our emotions. Breathing essential oils on a daily basis has helped me to release old negative emotions and replace them with positive, forward-moving thoughts and attitudes.

The more you use your oils in combination with prayer, the more you will see a shift in your mood, outlook, and thinking. Make the time for this to be a daily activity. Ask yourself how long you have had that negative emotion, release it, and give yourself time to heal. You are worth it. And once you release it, do not take it back.

Here are some other steps you can take:

+ Avoid the overuse of sugar and substances that depress your emotions.

+ Choose life-giving thoughts and life-giving habits that feed your emotional health.

+ Choose your friends wisely and avoid people who breed negativity and strife. Invest in positive relationships that help you feel great.

+ Become that positive uplifting person for others.

+ Avoid isolation. You were never meant to do life alone. Spend time with positive, loving people.

+ Began anointing and praying for others.

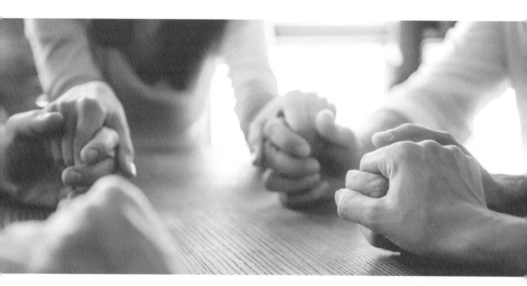

Pray and Anoint One Another

Anointing with precious oils and praying for each other is meant to be a common, everyday activity among loved ones. This is God's provision for us to live the abundant and healthy life He intends for us.

This activity will help you incorporate what you've been learning in this book. It starts in your daily life. With family, friends, or new acquaintances, be aware if someone is struggling. They may just be tired, weary from their job, or feeling discouraged. Maybe they are losing hope in some area.

At those times in my own life when I am struggling and need prayer, I don't lead in prayer for others; rather, I ask for prayer. Don't beat yourself up if you're not feeling strong enough to lead prayers. You will have seasons of giving and seasons of receiving. Be sensitive to yourself and ask for what you need.

When you are gathered with other people and someone is hurting, this is an opportunity to "bear one another's burdens" by praying for them and loving on them. If there is someone in the room who is full of faith and eager to pray, let them anoint with oil and pray with authority. It is always God who does the healing. There is power in knowing our authority in Christ to pray for healing.

God knows the thoughts and intents of our hearts, but sometimes, our deepest emotions are obscured from us until we learn how to examine our own heart. There is power and freedom as we learn to open ourselves up, be vulnerable to the Lord, and share our thoughts and emotions with Him. As you take the time to get in touch with your emotions, you become very clear about the reasons why you need prayer.

Pass around the frankincense oil or another essential oil that feels right, putting a few drops in each person's palm to breathe. Allow people plenty of time for introspection, to get in touch with their hearts and examine their thoughts. Then, when you are ready, let the person praying know what you are believing for and they will pray and believe with you.

This is a very sacred time. There should not be any distractions; everyone should be quiet and respectful of those being prayed for. Allow plenty of time for the Lord to move in this anointing; do not be in hurry.

We have seen many answered prayers during these times. Praying and expecting breakthrough requires faith—and taking a leap of faith can be scary. It may feel like you're jumping off a bridge and have no idea where you're going to land.

Before he became king, David had to deal with relentless assassination attempts instigated by King Saul. Yet he came to a place where he could look back and remember all of the times God had rescued him and focus on that. Those memories built his faith.

*I would have lost heart, unless I had believed that I would see the good-
ness of the L*ORD *in the land of the living.*   (Psalm 27:13 NKJV)

When you are up against a wall and struggling to keep your faith, go
back to a time in your life when you saw the evidence of God rescuing you
and hold on to that thought. Faith opens us to healing. Jesus delights when
we trust in Him and desires to pour out His healing grace.

*Then Jesus said to her, "Woman, you have great **faith**! Your request is
granted." And her daughter was healed at that moment.*

(Matthew 15:28)

*"Go," said Jesus, "your **faith** has healed you." Immediately he received
his sight and followed Jesus along the road.*

(Mark 10:52; see also Luke 18:42)

*As Jesus was on his way, the crowds almost crushed him. And a wom-
an was there who had been subject to bleeding for twelve years, but no
one could heal her. She came up behind him and touched the edge of
his cloak, and immediately her bleeding stopped. "Who touched me?"
Jesus asked.... Then the woman, seeing that she could not go unno-
ticed, came trembling and fell at his feet. In the presence of all the people, she told why she had touched him and how she had been instantly
healed. Then he said to her, "Daughter, your **faith** has healed you. Go
in peace."*   (Luke 8:42–45, 47–48)

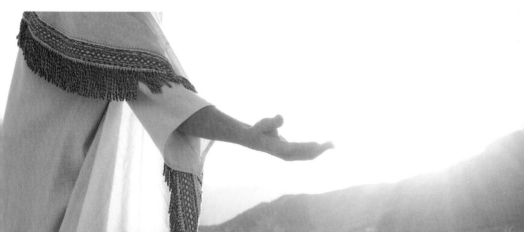

What a terrific story of faith! This woman had so much faith that she knew if she could just touch Jesus's garment, His love and healing would instantly cure her. If you're struggling with faith, start with gratitude.

Check out what Jeremiah says about God's absolute desire for you to live in health:

Behold, I will bring to it health and healing, and I will heal them; and I will reveal to them an abundance of peace and truth.

(Jeremiah 33:6 NASB)

Gratitude Opens the Floodgate to Healing

In my own personal journey to healthy emotions, I had to overcome a lot of anger and disappointment directed at God. When we lost our mom and sister at such a young age, I felt a lingering anger toward God for many months. Before their accident, I dreamed about what it would be like to get married and have children, knowing they would have the most wonderful grandparents. I thought about all the exciting adventures we would have "doing life" together. But I felt it had all been ripped away from me.

Then one day, I heard the Lord whisper to me, "Teri, you have the wrong perspective." I thought, *No, I don't. I have exactly the right perspective!* "No," He gently replied, "you are forgetting something very important. You had a loving mother for twenty-seven years and a best friend in your sister during your whole life. Many people around you never experienced the joy of a mother who loved them well, or a sister who loved them well."

Suddenly, I burst into tears. I was so ashamed of myself! I had become so self-absorbed that I had no sense of gratitude for all of the good years I had with my mom and sister, or the goodness of God that had surrounded us. All I could see was what I had lost.

From that day forward, I have always tried to examine my motives, my perspective, and my heart using essential oils to support my journey and release emotions I was struggling to let go of. I learned that it really does *not* matter what happens in life; it matters what we *think* about what happens to us. If you try hard enough, you will find something to be grateful for. Finding just one thing and focusing on that leads to one more thing…and one more thing. Gratitude ultimately opens a floodgate of healing balm to your soul and opens up streams of goodness that flow back to you. He came to give you an extravagant life, a life of meaning and joy.

We Are Designed for Joy

Joy is your birthright! Jesus taught us to pray, "*Your kingdom come, your will be done, on earth as it is in heaven*" (Matthew 6:10). Friend, there is no sickness in heaven, nor is there any sorrow or poverty. If we do the Father's will, we can bring heaven to earth—and that includes joy.

We are meant to live a fragrant, beautiful, healthy life. Adam and Eve were not placed in a sterile, bare home, but in a beautiful garden surrounded by fragrance and all of God's bountiful provision. So, let's begin to fully enjoy the scent of heaven that God has given to us.

Let all who take refuge in you be glad; let them ever sing for ***joy***.
(Psalm 5:11)

You will go out in ***joy*** *and be led forth in peace; the mountains and hills will burst into song before you, and all the trees of the field will clap their hands.* (Isaiah 55:12)

Ask and you will receive, and your ***joy*** *will be complete.* (John 16:24)

The Depths of Our Father's Love

Remember, God loves you with an extravagant love that can never be shaken. You may disappoint yourself or others, or even feel like you let God down, but His love is boundless. We need to bring our disappointments, especially with ourselves, directly to God and rediscover His love and forgiveness. When we fully embrace Him, there is no room left for fear, regret, or disappointment. Imagine that: the Creator of the universe loves you so deeply and tenderly that when you give Him the slightest attention, He is overwhelmed with joy.

God does everything for our good with lavish intent. He holds nothing back from us in terms of His love and His provision for our joy and our health. The plant oils He gave us to feed our body, nourish our soul, and make our spirit soar give us more evidence of God's extravagant provision for us to live a vibrant, healthy life. Everything that He placed in the garden of Eden for Adam and Eve to live life to the fullest is available to you. May God's gift of life and love be yours today—all of it!

With gratitude and enormous love,
Teri Secrest

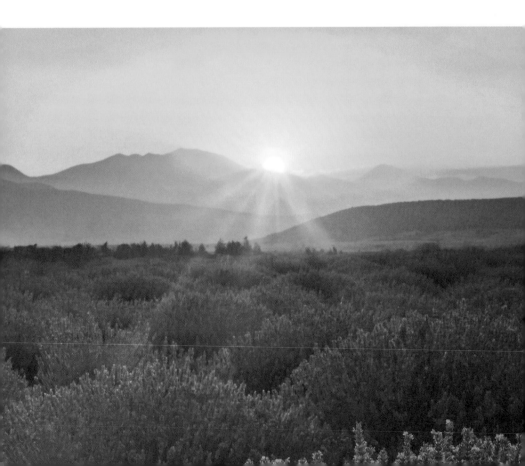

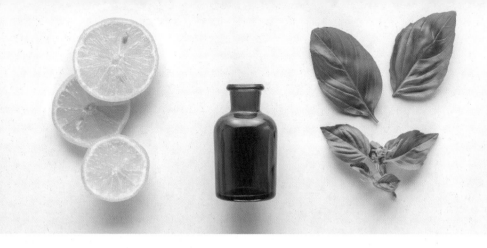

GLOSSARY

Carrier oil – an oil that can be used to dilute an essential oil so that it can be applied topically without adverse side effects; common carrier oils include olive, coconut, almond, avocado, flaxseed, and grapeseed

Diffuser – this device dispenses essential oil into the air as a fine mist or vapor

Iaomai – instantaneous healing

Supplement-grade essential oil – oil that's grown without the use of pesticides or herbicides, distilled at a low temperature, contains 100 percent essential oil (no additives), and is certified for internal use in small amounts per the label

Therapeutic-grade essential oil – oil that's grown without the use of pesticides or herbicides, distilled at a low temperature, contains 100 percent essential oil (no additives), and is labeled GRAS (Generally Regarded as Safe)

Therapeuo – gradual healing

Universal essential oil – one that supports nearly every system of the body

COME TO ME, ALL YOU WHO ARE WEARY AND
BURDENED, AND I WILL GIVE YOU REST.

—MATTHEW 11:28

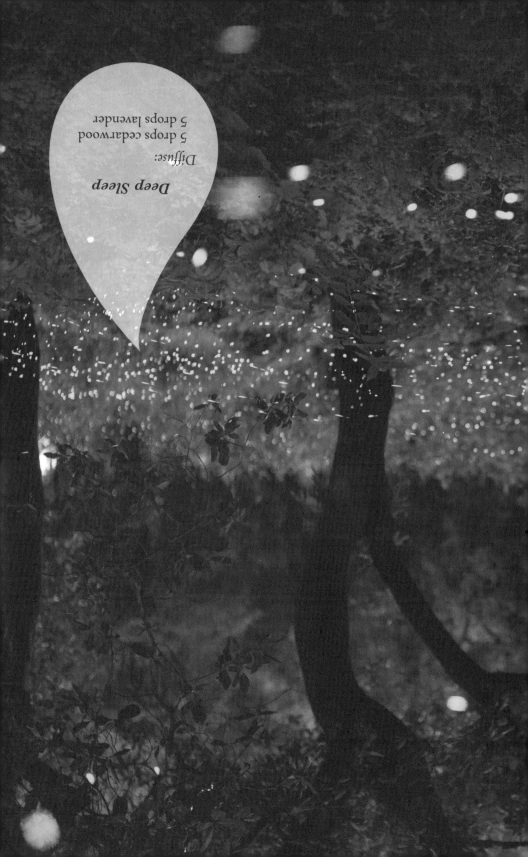

Deep Sleep

Diffuse:
5 drops cedarwood
5 drops lavender

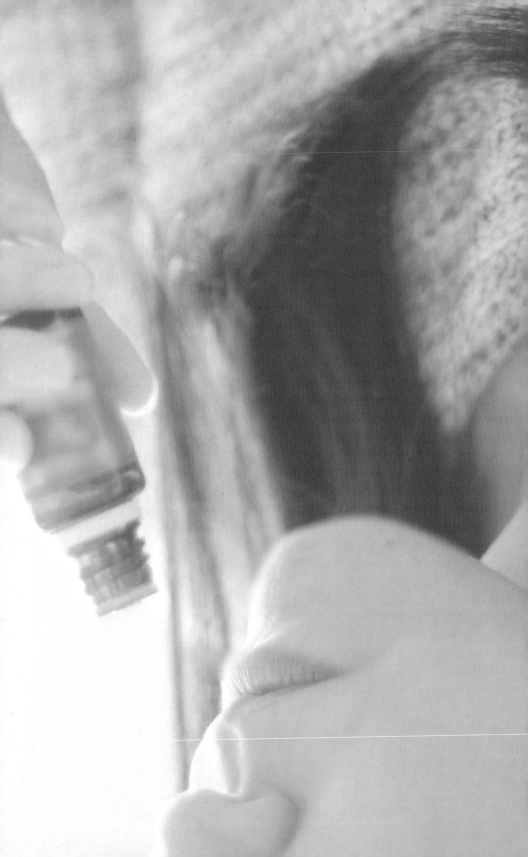

ESSENTIAL OILS
REFERENCE GUIDE

Please check with your doctor before starting any regimen of essential oils. Olive oil or coconut oil are beneficial for diluting essential oils that are "hot" on the skin, such as cinnamon, oregano, thyme, and cassia. The information provided herein is for educational purposes only and is not meant to diagnose or treat any condition.

Balsam Fir – stress, emotional unbalance, muscle tenseness

Basil – high cholesterol, poor cardiovascular system, unhealthy urinary system

Bergamot – high cholesterol, high blood pressure, fast heart rate, unbalanced hormones, emotional stress

Black Pepper – low libido

Blue Cypress – mental stress, brain fog

Calamus – muscle tenseness, depression, convulsions, pain

Cassia – emotional upset, tiredness, poor immune system, digestive problems

Cedarwood – brain fog, memory issues, ADHD, insomnia, hair loss, damaged hair, anxiety, congestion, skin issues or acne, respiratory problems, damaged bronchial tubes

Chamomile – inflamed joints, sore tendons; *in men*, high cortisol hormone levels

Cinnamon – common cold, poor cardiovascular system, digestive problems, unhealthy blood sugar levels, dental cavities, stress, tenseness, brain fog, urinary tract support

Cistus – congestion, phlegm, mucus

Citrus (Lemon, Orange, Tangerine, Grapefruit, Lime) – common cold, congestion, emotional upset, joint pain/stiffness, poor immune system, heartburn, unhealthy liver, stress

Clary Sage – high cortisol levels, stress; *in women*, unbalanced thyroid/hormone levels, low libido, vaginal dryness

Clove – common cold, tooth pain, diabetic neuropathy, unhealthy bladder

Cypress – skin issues/acne, poor blood circulation, excess fluid retention, respiratory problems

Eucalyptus – common cold

Eucalyptus Radiata – respiratory problems, damaged trachea

Frankincense – stress, congestion, inability to concentrate, skin issues/acne, damaged hair, respiratory problems, poor immune system, bacteria in the air, common cold, sunburn, unhealthy pituitary gland, gum inflammation, poor lymphatic system, sore muscles/tendons, poor nerve regeneration, unbalanced hormones/thyroids, anxiety; *in men*, low sperm count

Please check with your doctor before starting any regimen of essential oils.
Olive oil or coconut oil are beneficial for diluting essential oils that are "hot" on the skin,
such as cinnamon, oregano, thyme, and cassia. The information provided herein is for educational
purposes only and is not meant to diagnose or treat any condition.

Galbanum – skin issues/acne, anger

Geranium – nerve pain/injury, emotional stress/unbalance; *in women*, unhealthy estrogen or progesterone levels, unbalanced hormones, unhealthy reproductive system

Ginger – poor blood circulation, nausea, joint pain/stiffness, low libido

Goldenrod – *in men*, low libido, impotence

Helichrysum – poor immune system, high blood pressure, broken bones, sore muscles/tendons, poor nerve regeneration

Hyssop – respiratory problems, spasms, cough, sore throat, infection in small wounds, plaque formation from genital herpes, swollen ankles, hemorrhoids, poor blood circulation, digestive problems (indigestion, nausea, loss of appetite, heartburn, colic, gas), skin issues/acne, poor immune system, fever, phlegm, unhealthy urinary system

Jasmine – low libido

Juniper – poor blood circulation, muscle spasms, poor nerve regeneration

Lavender – stress, insomnia, unhealthy sleep patterns, restless legs, allergies, headache, skin issues/acne, burns, anger, agitation, anxiety, damaged hair, hypertension

Lemongrass – unhealthy/unbalanced thyroid gland, joint swelling/stiffness, sore muscles, weak ligaments/tissue, poor nervous system

Marjoram – tight/tense muscles, tendonitis, unhealthy urinary system

Please check with your doctor before starting any regimen of essential oils.
Olive oil or coconut oil are beneficial for diluting essential oils that are "hot" on the skin,
such as cinnamon, oregano, thyme, and cassia. The information provided herein is for educational
purposes only and is not meant to diagnose or treat any condition.

Myrrh (Stacte) – stress, poor immune system, skin issues/acne, gum disease, inflammation, common cold, small wounds, poor lymphatic system

Myrtle – skin issues/acne, hemorrhoids, congestion; *in women*, irregular menstrual cycle

Northern Lights Black Spruce – *in men*, low testosterone

Onycha – stress, tenseness, emotional repression, digestive problems, unhealthy blood sugar levels, germs/pollution in the air

Oregano – poor immune system, swollen lymph nodes, unhealthy urinary tract

Peppermint – tiredness, congestion, hunger, digestive problems, irritable bowel syndrome, broken bones, swollen lymph nodes, sore muscles, stomach ache, brain fog, memory issues; *in women*, hot flashes

Ravensara – respiratory problems

Rose – skin issues/acne; *in women*, low libido, vaginal dryness; *in men*, low sperm count, sexual dysfunction, performance anxiety

Rosemary – common cold, damaged hair, memory issues, unhealthy blood sugar levels, stress, muscle pain/inflammation, unhealthy urinary system, brain fog, discontentment; *in men*, high levels of estrogen

Rosewood – stress

Sage – unhealthy urinary system

Sandalwood – skin issues/acne, low libido, anxiety; *in men*, low testosterone levels

Spearmint – unhealthy parathyroid glands

Spikenard (Nard) – skin issues/acne, hair loss, damaged hair

Spruce – respiratory problems, weak bronchial tubes; *in men*, low testosterone

Tarragon – excess water retention

Tea Tree (Melaleuca) – infection in small wounds

Vanilla – emotional upset, stress

Vetiver – symptoms of ADHD

Wintergreen – broken bones, sore/tense muscles, congestion, respiratory problems

Ylang-ylang – irregular heartbeat, unbalanced hormones, low libido, unhealthy reproductive organs

Please check with your doctor before starting any regimen of essential oils.
Olive oil or coconut oil are beneficial for diluting essential oils that are "hot" on the skin,
such as cinnamon, oregano, thyme, and cassia. The information provided herein is for educational
purposes only and is not meant to diagnose or treat any condition.

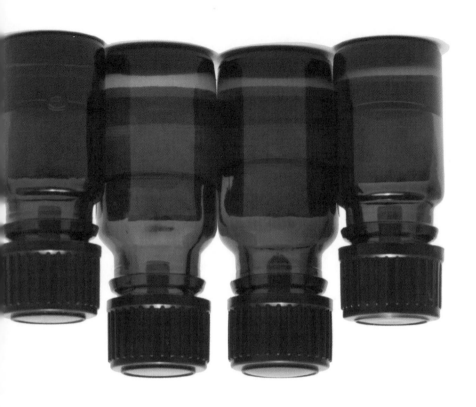

HEALTH CONCERNS AND HELPFUL ESSENTIAL OILS

Please check with your doctor before starting any regimen of essential oils. Olive oil or coconut oil are beneficial for diluting essential oils that are "hot" on the skin, such as cinnamon, oregano, thyme, and cassia. The information provided herein is for educational purposes only and is not meant to diagnose or treat any condition.

Cardiovascular/Circulatory System	helichrysum, cypress, lemon
Balance Blood Sugar Levels	cinnamon, onycha, coriander
Fast Heart Rate	bergamot
High Blood Pressure	bergamot, helichrysum
High Cholesterol	basil, bergamot
Hypertension	lavender
Irregular Heartbeat	ylang-ylang
Poor Blood Circulation	cypress, ginger, hyssop, juniper

Digestive System	cassia, cinnamon, hyssop, onycha, peppermint
Colic	hyssop
Excess Fluid Retention	cypress, tarragon
Heartburn	citrus (lemon, orange, tangerine, grapefruit, lime), hyssop
Hemorrhoids	hyssop, myrtle
Hunger	peppermint
Irritable Bowel Syndrome	peppermint
Liver Support	citrus (lemon, orange, tangerine, grapefruit, lime)
Nausea	ginger, hyssop
Stomach Ache	peppermint

Endocrine/Reproductive Systems	geranium, ylang-ylang
High Cortisol Hormone Levels	clary sage; *in men*, chamomile
High Levels of Estrogen	*in men*, rosemary
Hot Flashes	peppermint
Irregular Menstrual cycle	myrtle
Low Libido	black pepper, ginger, jasmine, sandalwood, ylang-ylang; *in women*, clary sage, rose; *in men*, goldenrod
Low Sperm Count *in men*	frankincense, rose
Low Testosterone Levels *in men*	northern lights black spruce, sandalwood, spruce
Sexual Dysfunction/Impotence	frankincense, goldenrod, rose
Unbalanced Hormones/Thyroid	bergamot, frankincense, lemongrass, ylang-ylang; *in women*, clary sage, geranium
Unhealthy Estrogen or Progesterone Levels *in women*	geranium
Unhealthy Parathyroid Glands	spearmint
Unhealthy Pituitary Gland	frankincense
Vaginal Dryness *in women*	clary sage, rose

Please check with your doctor before starting any regimen of essential oils.
Olive oil or coconut oil are beneficial for diluting essential oils that are "hot" on the skin,
such as cinnamon, oregano, thyme, and cassia. The information provided herein is for educational
purposes only and is not meant to diagnose or treat any condition.

Immune System	cassia, frankincense, helichrysum, hyssop, myrrh, oregano
Common Cold	cinnamon, citrus (lemon, orange, tangerine, grapefruit, lime), clove, eucalyptus, frankincense, myrrh, rosemary
Congestion	cedarwood, citrus (lemon, orange, tangerine, grapefruit, lime), frankincense, hyssop, peppermint, wintergreen
Fever	hyssop, peppermint
Sore Throat	hyssop

Integumentary System	
Hair Loss/Damaged Hair	cedarwood, frankincense, lavender, rosemary, spikenard
Skin Issues/Acne	cedarwood, cypress, frankincense, galbanum, hyssop, lavender, myrrh, myrtle, rose, sandalwood, spikenard
Sunburn/Burns	frankincense, lavender

Please check with your doctor before starting any regimen of essential oils.
Olive oil or coconut oil are beneficial for diluting essential oils that are "hot" on the skin,
such as cinnamon, oregano, thyme, and cassia. The information provided herein is for educational
purposes only and is not meant to diagnose or treat any condition.

Lymphatic System	cypress, frankincense, myrrh
Swollen Lymph Nodes	cypress, oregano, peppermint

Mental Health	
ADHD	cedarwood, vetiver
Anger	galbanum, lavender
Anxiety	cedarwood, frankincense, lavender, sandalwood
Brain Fog	blue cypress, cedarwood, cinnamon, frankincense, peppermint, rosemary
Discontentment	rosemary
Emotional Stress	balsam fir, bergamot, calamus, cassia, citrus (lemon, orange, tangerine, grapefruit, lime), geranium, onycha, vanilla
Insomnia	cedarwood, lavender
Memory Issues	cedarwood, peppermint, rosemary
Stress	balsam fir, blue cypress, citrus (lemon, orange, tangerine, grapefruit, lime), clary sage, frankincense, lavender, myrrh, onycha, rosemary, rosewood, vanilla
Tiredness	cassia, peppermint

Please check with your doctor before starting any regimen of essential oils.
Olive oil or coconut oil are beneficial for diluting essential oils that are "hot" on the skin,
such as cinnamon, oregano, thyme, and cassia. The information provided herein is for educational
purposes only and is not meant to diagnose or treat any condition.

Miscellaneous

Allergies	lavender
Dental Cavities	myrrh
Germs/Bacteria in the Air	frankincense, onycha
Gum Disease/Inflammation	frankincense, myrrh
Headache	lavender
Small Wounds	hyssop, myrrh, tea tree
Tooth Ache	clove, myrrh

Nervous System — lemongrass

Nerve Pain/Injury	geranium, juniper
Numbness and Tingling	nutmeg, cypress
Poor Nerve Regeneration	frankincense, helichrysum, juniper

Respiratory System — cedarwood, cistus, cypress, eucalyptus radiata, frankincense, hyssop, ravensara, spruce, wintergreen

Cough	hyssop
Bronchial Support	cedarwood, spruce
Trachea Support	eucalyptus radiata

Please check with your doctor before starting any regimen of essential oils.
Olive oil or coconut oil are beneficial for diluting essential oils that are "hot" on the skin,
such as cinnamon, oregano, thyme, and cassia. The information provided herein is for educational
purposes only and is not meant to diagnose or treat any condition.

Skeletal/Muscular Systems

Broken Bones	helichrysum, peppermint, wintergreen
Convulsions/Spasms	lavender, hyssop, juniper
Inflammation	copaiba, frankincense, rosemary
Joint Pain/Stiffness/Swelling	chamomile, citrus (lemon, orange, tangerine, grapefruit, lime), ginger, hyssop, lemongrass
Muscle Pain/Stiffness/Swelling	balsam fir, calamus, cinnamon, frankincense, helichrysum, juniper, lemongrass, marjoram, onycha, peppermint, rosemary, wintergreen
Pain	wintergreen, peppermint, helichrysum, rosemary
Restless Legs	lavender
Sore Tendons	chamomile, frankincense, helichrysum
Tendonitis	marjoram
Weak Ligaments/Tissue	lemongrass

Please check with your doctor before starting any regimen of essential oils.
Olive oil or coconut oil are beneficial for diluting essential oils that are "hot" on the skin,
such as cinnamon, oregano, thyme, and cassia. The information provided herein is for educational
purposes only and is not meant to diagnose or treat any condition.

Urinary System	basil, cinnamon, hyssop, marjoram, oregano, rosemary, sage
Bladder Support	frankincense, juniper, oregano
Urinary Tract Infection	myrrh, mountain savory, oregano

Please check with your doctor before starting any regimen of essential oils.
Olive oil or coconut oil are beneficial for diluting essential oils that are "hot" on the skin,
such as cinnamon, oregano, thyme, and cassia. The information provided herein is for educational
purposes only and is not meant to diagnose or treat any condition.

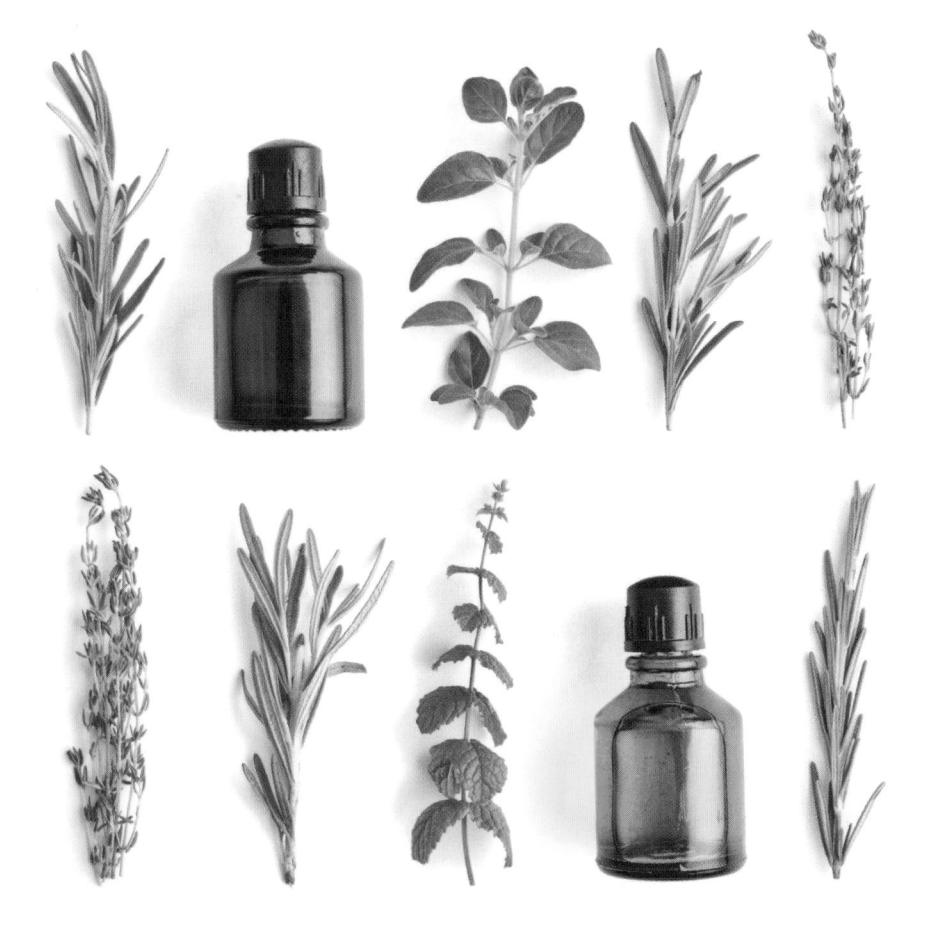

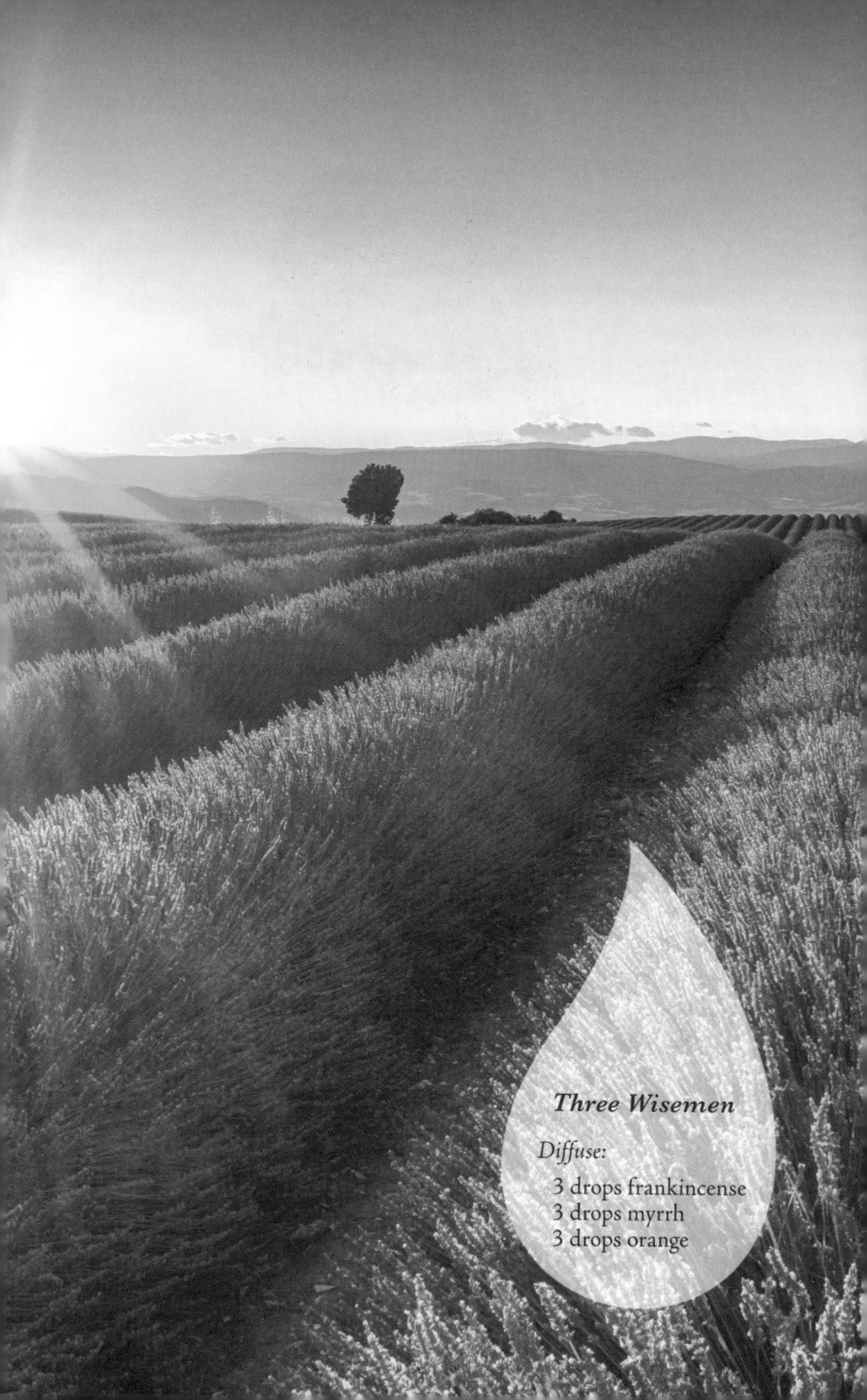

Three Wisemen

Diffuse:

3 drops frankincense
3 drops myrrh
3 drops orange

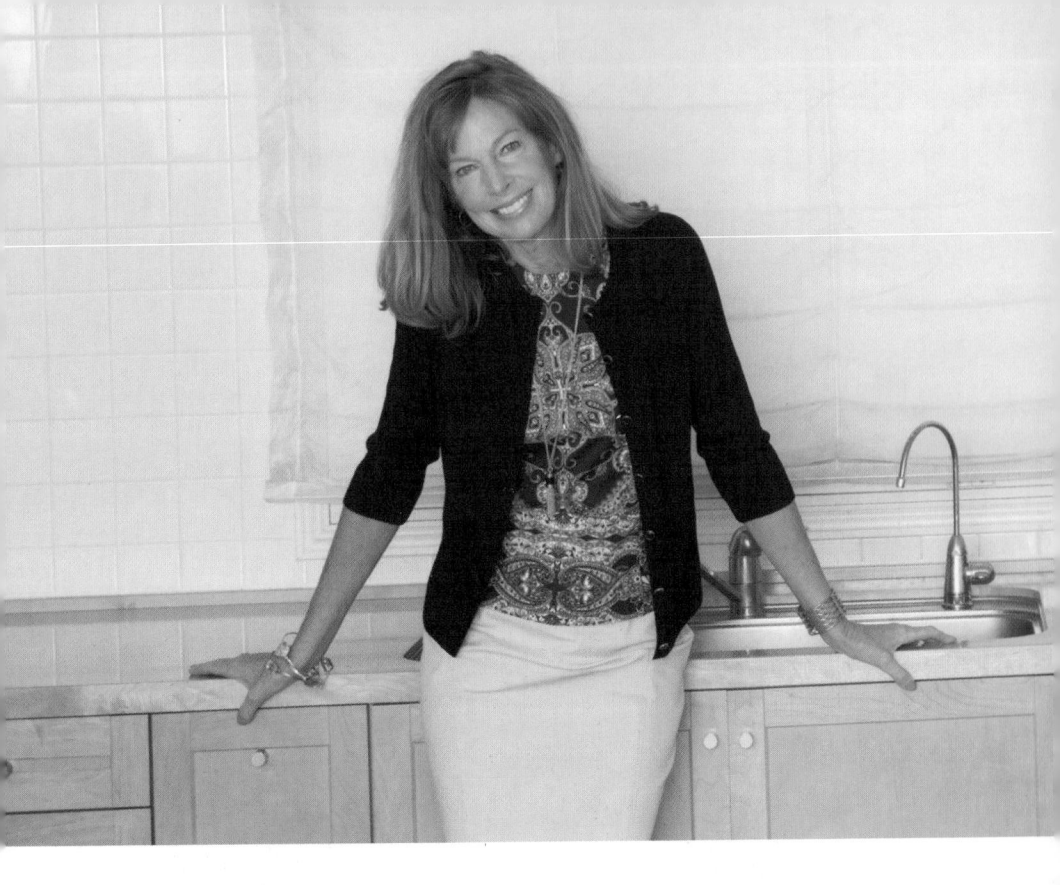

ABOUT THE AUTHOR

Teri Secrest is a health and wellness expert whose passion is to teach simple and proven methods for vibrant health to people around the world. That passion is rooted in her early experiences of learning about whole foods and herbs in her family's organic garden and her mother's love for good food as the owner of a French cooking school. These early lessons guided Teri to a healthy path for herself and her own family, yet it was her first astonishing experience with essential oils as a young mother that ignited her lifelong quest for learning, practicing, and teaching people to take hold of God's extravagant provision for their health.

Teri has traveled around the world to learn from leading experts about the beneficial uses of essential oils, research the promises and properties of

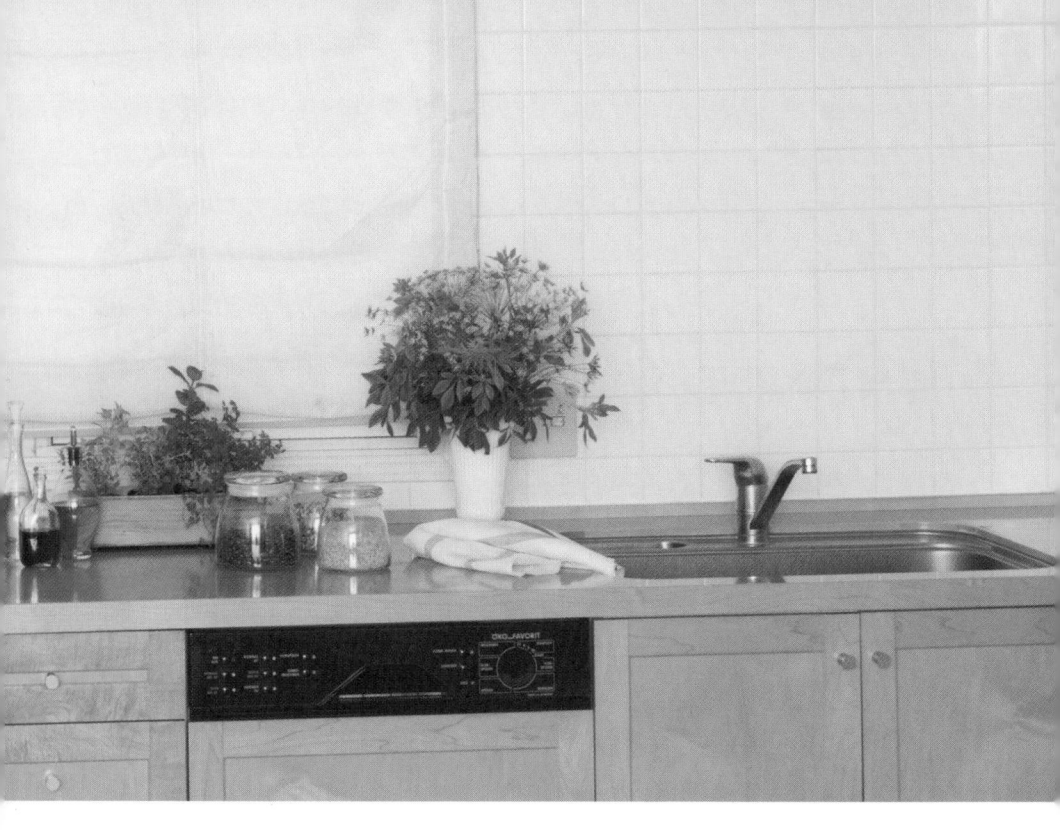

each essential oil, and develop a deep working knowledge of their applications for daily health and wellness.

Teri loves to share the simple, practical principles that will help you live in vibrant health through her international keynote speeches, training programs, and best-selling books. She is a sought-after speaker who delivers her message of vibrant health with such enthusiasm, humor, and joy that she has gained the nickname "Ambassador of Joy" around the world.

Connect with Teri:

http://terisecrest.com

https://www.facebook.com/TeriSecrestInternational

https://twitter.com/terisecrest

https://www.instagram.com/teri.secrest

https://www.youtube.com/TeriLeeSecrest

info@terisecrest.com

1-855-SECREST (732-7378)

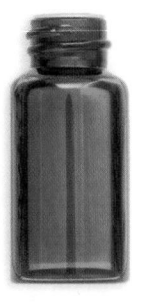

ENDNOTES
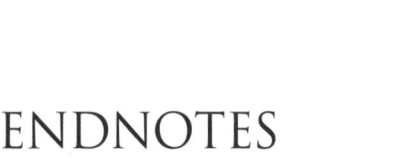

1. "Proportion and number of cancer cases and deaths attributable to potentially modifiable risk factors in the United States," *CA: A Cancer Journal for Clinicians*, November 21, 2017 (onlinelibrary.wiley.com/doi/full/10.3322/caac.21440).

2. "Nutrition, Physical Activity, and Obesity: Keeping Americans Healthy at Every Stage of Life," CDC (www.cdc.gov/chronicdisease/resources/publications/aag/pdf/2016/aag-dnpao.pdf).

3. CDC, *National Diabetes Statistics Report 2017* (www.cdc.gov/diabetes/data/statistics/statistics-report.html).

4. "Caloric Intake From Fast Food Among Children and Adolescents in the United States, 2011–2012," NCHS Data Brief, September 2015 (www.cdc.gov/nchs/products/databriefs/db213.htm).

5. "Fast-Food Habits, Weight Gain, and Insulin Resistance (the CARDIA Study): 15-year prospective analysis," *The Lancet*, January 2005 (www.researchgate.net/publication/8090990_Fast-Food_Habits_Weight_Gain_and_Insulin_Resistance_the_CARDIA_Study_15-year_prospective_analysis).

6. www.cdc.gov/obesity/index.html.

7. "Depression—A Global Public Health Concern," World Health Organization 2012 report, (www.who.int/mental_health/management/depression/who_paper_depression_wfmh_2012.pdf).

8. "Antidepressant Use Among Persons Aged 12 and Over: United States, 2011–2014," CDC, National Center for Health Statistics (NCHS) Data Brief, August 2017 (www.cdc.gov/nchs/data/databriefs/db283.pdf).

9. Jennifer Billock, "Explore the Ruins of an Ancient Incense Route," *Smithsonian Magazine*, January 26, 2017 (www.smithsonianmag.com/travel/visit-remnants-ancient-incense-route-180961873).

10. "Essential oil," *New World Encyclopedia* (www.newworldencyclopedia.org/entry/Essential_oil).

11. Chelsea R. Manion and Rebecca M. Widder, "Essentials of essential oils," *American Journal of Health-System Pharmacy*, Volume 74, Issue 9, May 1, 2017 (academic.oup.com/ajhp/article/74/9/e153/5102762).

12. www.fda.gov/consumers/consumer-updates/combating-antibiotic-resistance.

13. Stevie Wonder, "Don't You Worry 'bout a Thing," on *Innervisions* (Tamla, 1974).

14. www.humanolfaction.org.

15. David Stewart, *Healing Oils of the Bible* (Marble Hill, MO: Napsac International, 2004).

16. "Effect of myrrh oil on IL-1β stimulation of NF-ᴋB activation and PGE2 production in human gingival fibroblasts and epithelial cells," *Toxicology in Vitro*, Volume 20, Issue 2, March 2006 (see Abstract, www.sciencedirect.com/science/article/pii/S0887233305001554); "Evaluation of the Antibacterial Efficacy of Azadirachta Indica, Commiphora Myrrha, Glycyrrhiza Glabra Against Enterococcus Faecalis using Real Time PCR," *The Open Dentistry Journal*, Vol. 10, 2016 (opendentistryjournal.com/VOLUME/10/PAGE/160).

17. "In Vitro Anti-Cariogenic Plaque Effects of Essential Oils Extracted from Culinary Herbs," Current Neurology and Neuroscience Reports, September 2017 (www.ncbi.nlm.nih.gov/pubmed/29207708).

18. Gary Young, *Essential Oils Desk Reference 6th ed.* (Lehi, UT: Life Science Publishing, 2014).

19. David Stewart, *The Chemistry of Essential Oils Made Simple: God's Love Manifest in Molecules* (Marble Hill, MO: Care Publications, 2013).

20. Herbert Baxter and Jeffrey Harborne, *Chemical Dictionary of Economic Plants* (Somerset, NJ: J. Wiley & Sons, 2001).

21. Jennifer Peace Rhind, *Essential Oils: A Handbook for Aromatherapy Practice* (London, UK: Singing Dragon, 2012).

22. K. G. Stiles, *The Essential Oils Complete Reference Guide: Over 250 Recipes for Natural Wholesome Aromatherapy* (Salem, MA: Page Street Publishing Co., 2017).

23. Milica Ljaljević Grbić et al, "Frankincense and myrrh essential oils and burn incense fume against micro-inhabitants of sacral ambients. Wisdom of the ancients?," *Journal of Ethnopharmacology*, Vol. 219, June 12, 2018 (www.sciencedirect.com/science/article/pii/S0378874117342745).

24. "Frankincense's Efficacy in Treating Osteoarthritis," *Natural Medicine Journal*, May 2013 (www.naturalmedicinejournal.com/journal/2013-05/frankincenses-efficacy-treating-osteoarthritis).

25. John C. Maxwell, *The Maxwell Leadership Bible: Lessons in Leadership from the Word of God* (Nashville, TN: Thomas Nelson, 2014).

26. Robert Jamieson, A.R. Fausset, and David Brown, "Commentary on Esther 2:12," *Commentary Critical and Explanatory on the Whole Bible – Unabridged*, 1871-1878 (www.studylight.org/commentaries/jfu/esther-2.html).

27. enduringword.com/bible-commentary/song-of-solomon-5.

28. Milica Ljaljević Grbić et al.

29. files.meetup.com/1481956/ADHD%20Research%20by%20Dr.%20Terry%20Friedmann.pdf.

30. "Susceptibility of Drug-Resistant Clinical Herpes Simplex Virus Type 1 Strains to Essential Oils of Ginger, Thyme, Hyssop, and Sandalwood," *Antimicrobial Agents and Chemotherapy*, March 12, 2007 (www.ncbi.nlm.nih.gov/pmc/articles/PMC1855548).

31. Kiran Patil, "17 Best Benefits of Hyssop Essential Oil," *Organic Facts*, March 2019 (www.organicfacts.net/health-benefits/essential-oils/health-benefits-of-hyssop-essential-oil.html).

32. Cathy Wong, "Health Benefits of Rose Essential Oil," *Very Well Health*, March 2019 (www.verywellhealth.com/the-benefits-of-rose-essential-oil-88790).

33. "Randomized Trial of Aromatherapy; Successful Treatment for Alopecia Areata," *Archives of Dermatology*, Vol. 134, No. 11, November 1, 1998 (jamanetwork.com/journals/jamadermatology/article-abstract/189618).

34. organic.org/healing-herbs-for-the-respiratory-system.

35. "Anti-inflammatory and antioxidant properties of Helichrysum italicum," The Journal of Pharmacy and Pharmacology, April 2002 (www.researchgate.net/publication/11460837_ Anti-inflammatory_and_antioxidant_ properties_of_Helichrysum_italicum).

36. "Frankincense (Rû Xiãng; Boswellia Species): From the Selection of Traditional Applications to the Novel Phytotherapy for the Prevention and Treatment of Serious Diseases," *Journal of Traditional and Complementary Medicine*, Oct.-Dec. 2013 (www.ncbi. nlm.nih.gov/pmc/articles/PMC3924999).

37. "Bergamot Extract May Lower Your Cholesterol; Statin dose cut with citrus fruit," *Health Essentials* from Cleveland Clinic, May 6, 2015 (health.clevelandclinic.org/bergamot-may-lower-your-cholesterol).

38. "Aromatherapy Benefits Autonomic Nervous System Regulation for Elementary School Faculty in Taiwan," *Advances in Decision Sciences*, April 10, 2011, (www.hindawi.com/ journals/ecam/2011/946537).

39. "Effect of fibre, antispasmodics, and peppermint oil in the treatment of irritable bowel syndrome: systematic review and meta-analysis," *British Medical Journal*, Nov. 13, 2008 (www.ncbi.nlm.nih.gov/pmc/articles/PMC2583392/?tool=pubmed).

40. "Ginger for nausea and vomiting of pregnancy," Canadian Family Physician, February 2016 (www.ncbi.nlm.nih.gov/pmc/articles/PMC4755634).

41. "An Experimental Study on the Effectiveness of Massage with Aromatic Ginger and Orange Essential Oil for Moderate-to-Severe Knee Discomfort among the Elderly in Hong Kong," *Complementary Therapies in Medicine*, June 2008 (www.ncbi.nlm.nih.gov/ pubmed/18534325).

42. "The effect of Frankincense in the treatment of moderate plaque-induced gingivitis: a double blinded randomized clinical trial," *Daru: Journal of Faculty of Pharmacy*, Tehran University of Medical Sciences, 2011 (www.ncbi.nlm.nih.gov/pmc/articles/PMC3304380).

43. Cindy Jones, "Protect Your Bones with Herbs: Recent study shows common herbs help decrease osteoporosis risk," *Mother Earth Living*, March/April 2004 (www. motherearthliving.com/health-and-wellness/protec-your-bones-with-herbs).

44. "Effects of Eugenol on Nerve and Vascular Dysfunction in Streptozotocin-Diabetic Rats," *Planta Medica*, 2006 (www.thieme-connect.com/products/ejournals/ html/10.1055/s-2005-916262).

45. "The acute airway inflammation induced by PM2.5 exposure and the treatment of essential oils in Balb/c mice," *Scientific Reports*, March 9, 2017 (www.ncbi.nlm.nih.gov/pmc/ articles/PMC5343586).

46. "Effect of Essential Oils on Pathogenic Bacteria," *Pharmaceuticals*, Nov. 25, 2013 (www. mdpi.com/1424-8247/6/12/1451/htm).

47. "Frankincense (Rû Xiãng; Boswellia Species); see 38.

48. William Dufty, *Sugar Blues* (Padnor, PA: Chilton Book Co., 1975).

49. Teri Secrest, *Eating Out of Heaven's Garden* (Lehi, UT: Life Science Publishing, 2012).

50. Tim and Beverly LaHaye, *The Act of Marriage: The Beauty of Sexual Love* (Grand Rapids, MI: Zondervan, 1976).

51. Gary Thomas, Cherish: The One Word That Changes Everything for Your Marriage (Grand Rapids, MI: Zondervan, 2017).

52. "Effects of Fragrance Inhalation on Sympathetic Activity in Normal Adults," *Japanese Journal of Pharmacology*, November 2002 (pdfs.semanticscholar.org/ e47f/58f0996e7dd1a5aa90794f961e532aafdba5.pdf).

53. Margo Arrowsmith, "Norman Cousins: The Man Who Laughed In The Face of Death," *Remedy Grove*, November 16, 2017 (remedygrove.com/wellness/normancousins).

54. www.patchadams.org.

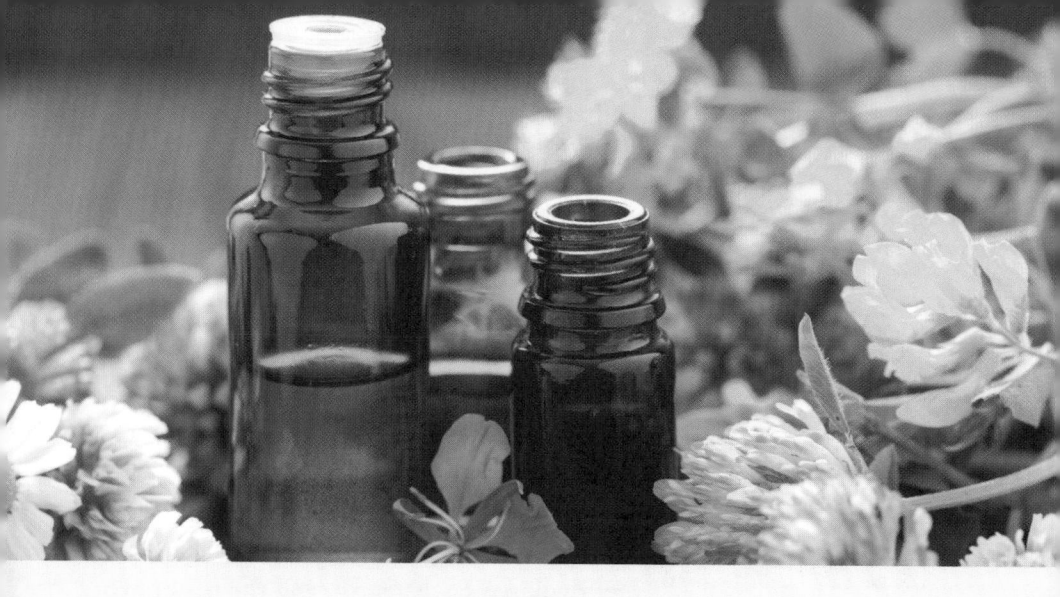

WHERE TO PURCHASE QUALITY ESSENTIAL OILS

As a certified wellness coach, I have had the privilege of living in Europe for five years and traveling around the world for the past 25 years, investigating essential oils.

If you have a good supplier of top-quality essential oils, please continue to honor that relationship. However, if you are looking for high-quality, supplement-grade essential oils, I invite you to contact our office at **info@terisecrest.com** or call the Essential Oils Healthline toll-free at **1-833-OIL-LINE (645-5463)**.

An exemplary essential oil company controls the entire life cycle of the plant from the planting to the harvesting, distillation, and bottling. The source plants, flowers, and trees are grown in healthy soil without pesticides or herbicides; harvested precisely at their peak; either cold-pressed or steam distilled at low temperatures to preserve their therapeutic value; and carefully sealed in dark bottles. Every step is managed with the utmost care to preserve the delicate, health-supporting capabilities of the essential oils.

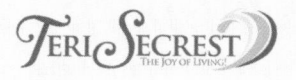

A Biblical Perspective on Essential Oils

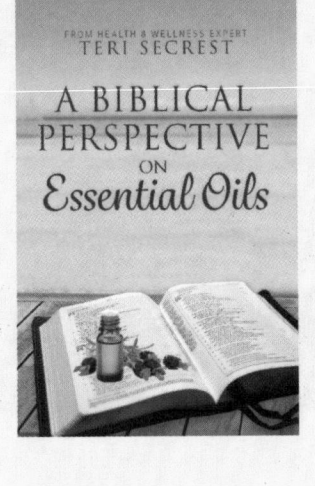

Booklet: full color, 48 pages

After 25 years of study, practical application, and research, Teri Secrest shares her world-changing teaching—*A Biblical Perspective on Essential Oils*! Join Teri on this intriguing journey through history to learn the secret to Queen Esther's beauty, the wisdom about health that King Solomon imparted to all the kings of the earth, and the reason that Moses continued to walk in strength all during his later years! Find out how to apply this same wisdom today to enjoy maximum joy and vitality in your life! This booklet is a perfect tool to use for a small group training.

Eating Out of Heaven's Garden

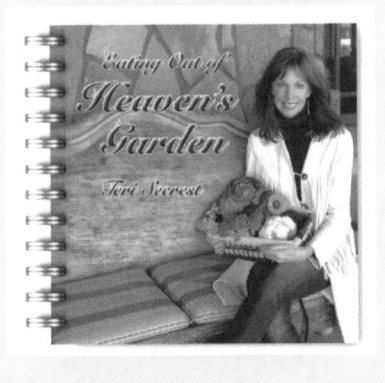

Book: full color, spiral bound, 152 pages

Your love affair with food has just begun! Teri Secrest is passionate about delicious, healthy food. As the daughter of a French chef, Teri learned the power of a colorful, nutrition- filled diet when she was very young. This love has taken her all over the world, teaching vibrant health and longevity.

If you are ready to kick the junk-food lifestyle, this book is for you! Over ninety pages of delicious recipes, many from Teri's own kitchen! Learn how to add extra zest and nutrition to recipes with supplement-grade essential oils. *Eating Out of Heaven's Garden* makes eating healthy, delicious, and full of joy.

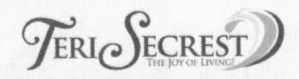

These and other great resources are available at TeriSecrest.com